A Mixed Bag

An enquiry into the care of hospital patients receiving parenteral nutrition

A report by the National Confidential Enquiry into Patient Outcome and Death (2010)

Written by:

J A D Stewart MB ChB LLM FRCP
Clinical Co-ordinator

D G Mason MBBS FFARCS
Clinical Co-ordinator

N Smith PhD
Clinical Researcher

K Protopapa BSc
Researcher

M Mason PhD
Chief Executive

The authors and Trustees of NCEPOD would particularly like to thank the NCEPOD staff for their work in collecting and analysing the data for this study:

Robert Alleway, Sabah Begg, Bryony Bull, Maurice Blackman, Heather Freeth, Dolores Jarman, Kathryn Kelly, Rakhee Lakhani, Waqaar Majid, Eva Nwosu and Hannah Shotton.

Contents

Acknowledgements

This report, published by NCEPOD, could not have been achieved without the support of a wide range of individuals who have contributed to this study.

Our particular thanks go to:

The expert group who advised NCEPOD on what to assess during this study:

Melanie Baker	Dietitian
Andrea Cartwright	Nutrition Nurse Specialist
Lynne Colagiovanni	Nurse Consultant in Nutrition Support
Angie Davidson	Nurse Consultant in Nutrition and Intestinal Failure
Kenny McCormick	Consultant Neonatologist
Simon McPherson	Consultant Radiologist and NCEPOD Steering Group member
Jeremy Nightingale	Consultant Gastroenterologist
Jeremy Powell-Tuck	Emeritus Professor of Clinical Nutrition
John Puntis	Consultant Paediatric Gastroenterologist
Jon Shaffer	Consultant Gastroenterologist
Carolyn Wheatley	Lay Representative – BAPEN
Rebecca White	Pharmacist

The Advisors who reviewed the cases:

Tariq Ahmad	Consultant Gastroenterologist
Peter Austin	Senior Pharmacist
Tim Bowling	Consultant Gastroenterologist
Helen Budge	Consultant Paediatric Gastroenterologist
Nicola Burch	Specialist Registrar in Gastroenterology
Pam Cairns	Consultant Neonatologist
David Campbell	Consultant Paediatric Gastroenterologist
Stanley Craig	Consultant Neonatologist
Sue Cullen	Consultant Gastroenterologist
Sarah Cunningham	Paediatric Nurse Specialist in Nutrition
Ieuan Davies	Consultant Paediatric Gastroenterologist
Jacqueline Eastwood	Senior Pharmacist
Nevine El-Sherbini	Dietitian
Nick Embleton	Consultant Neonatologist
Simon Fleming	Consultant in Clinical Biochemistry & Metabolic Medicine
Stephen Foley	Consultant Gastroenterologist
Emma Forsyth	Senior Specialist Dietitian
Donnay Gallinetti	Dietitian
Emma Greig	Consultant Gastroenterologist
Amit Gupta	Consultant Neonatologist
Claire Hamer	Dietitian
Susan Hill	Consultant Paediatric Gastroenterologist
Jonathan Hind	Consultant Paediatric Hepatology
Shorland Hosking	Consultant Surgeon

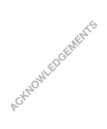

Richard Johnston	Gastroenterology Research Registrar
Amelia Jukes	Dietitian
Linda Kenny	Advanced Nurse Practitioner, Nutrition
Jamil Khair	Paediatric Clinical Nurse Specialist
Chris Langrish	Consultant Intensivist
Subramanian Mahadevan	Consultant Paediatrician
Clifford Mayes	Consultant Neonatologist
Judith McGovern	Nutrition Nurse Specialist
Nigel Meadows	Consultant Paediatric Gastroenterologist
Gopi Menon	Consultant Neonatologist
Vinita Mishra	Consultant Chemical Pathologist
Penny Neild	Consultant Gastroenterologist
Lindsay Newell	Dietitian
Louise Reissner	Dietitian
Joanne Sayer	Consultant Gastroenterologist
Julia Smith	Paediatric Gastroenterology Dietitian
Stephanie Strachan	Consultant Intensivist
Adrian Thomas	Consultant Paediatric Gastroenterologist
Sabita Uthaya	Consultant Neonatologist
Vimal Vasu	Consultant Neonatologist

Additional thanks go to Professor Martin Utley and Professor Steve Gallivan from the Clinical Operational Research Unit at University College London for their scientific advice.

Foreword

Despite various initiatives through professional bodies such as the British Association of Parenteral and Enteral Nutrition, there is a broad suspicion that nutrition is a serious problem within our hospitals. The introduction of the Malnutrition Universal Screening Tool (MUST), and the 'red tray' scheme have heightened awareness and are important interventions in the fight against Hospital Acquired Malnutrition. However, there has as yet been little proactive intervention in the area of parenteral nutrition (PN). This does not reflect an unwillingness to improve matters by the nutrition professionals and their representative bodies, but rather a lack of ammunition with which to show that matters need to be improved.

We think this report is the first national observational study on PN ever carried out in the UK and we hope it will go some way to persuade hospitals that it is time to hear the voice of the nutrition community when they demand that PN care be improved.

This report is a description of a random sample of all patients who were given PN over a given period of time. As such there is reason to suppose that it is representative of the care received by all such patients across the NHS. Because PN is an expensive and hazardous intervention it should only be adopted where it is necessary to sustain a patient who is recognised to be extremely ill or for treating premature neonates who have a very low nutritional reserve and immature gut function. Thus one might expect it would only be initiated after careful thought and carried out under close supervision. Certainly we hoped that this group would represent the NHS at its best.

It is thus deeply depressing that the advisors should have found that the quality of care is so often unsatisfactory. Indeed, in our debates within the multi-collegiate NCEPOD Steering Group the scale of disappointment verged on disbelief. We found that only 19% of the adult cohort could be said to represent good practice (see Table 2.1); that is the standard of care that the Advisors would accept from themselves, their trainees and their institutions. Neonates did only marginally better at 23.5% (Table 3.1).

The great strength of an observational study is that the advisors have free rein to pick out the real story, the important lessons that they believe can be drawn from the cases they have studied. We depend upon their opinions being fair. It is shocking that over half of the cases lacked an adequate clinical assessment of the patient's nutritional needs (Table 2.15); but it naturally follows that a similar proportion lacked any documentation of the patient's supposed nutritional requirements before the team started to deliver it parenterally (Table 2.16).

Another striking finding that the advisors identified was the variation in neonatal PN practice between units, particularly for extremely low birth weight neonates. Obtaining a greater consensus in best PN neonatal practice should be a priority for all those involved in the care of this group of patients.

If the spectre of malnutrition is to be banished from our wards, I suggest that a Nutrition Tsar could help to harness energies and ensure that everyone recognises that the nutritionists and dietitians have a contribution to make to the welfare of many patients and that in the case of this very sick group of people, that contribution is central to their medical care.

On behalf of the Trustees I would like to thank the Local Reporters, the clinicians who filled in their questionnaires, and those people within the Trusts who did produce the copies of notes, despite their scanty resources. Also the 11 members of the expert group who helped us to design the study; the 44 Advisors who reviewed the cases and whose assessments form the bedrock of this report; the staff, the authors and the Steering Group who have all done so much to produce this portrait of parenteral nutrition as it is delivered in the UK today. I commend it to you as a solid piece of work, even though it describes a disappointing state of affairs.

This challenge now is to use these important findings to make a significant difference to patient care in the future.

Bertie Leigh
Chair of NCEPOD

Introduction

The administration of parenteral nutrition (PN) is a well established technique providing nutritional support to patients who have an inaccessible or non-functioning gut (intestinal failure). As such it is widely used by surgeons, intensivists, paediatricians, neonatologists, oncologists and clinical nutrition specialists. However it is available to all clinicians regardless of specialty or expertise in its use. Whilst PN is undoubtedly a vital piece of the clinician's armoury, and a potential lifesaver, it can also be fraught with potentially fatal complications. Thus it should never be given without appropriate forethought and planning. For PN to be given safely it requires an accurate assessment of the patient's nutritional requirements, appropriate constitution and compounding of the PN, safe intravenous access (with meticulous aseptic insertion technique and subsequent catheter care) and rigorous monitoring of the patient's

electrolytes and anthropometric response. Ideally these parameters should be achieved through a co-ordinated team approach of clinicians, dietitians, nutrition nurse specialists and pharmacists; preferably operating within a nutrition team and working with appropriately trained and experienced clinical ward staff. This approach has been broadly reflected by the British Association of Parenteral and Enteral Nutrition through their OFNoSH initiative.[1] However, the extent to which this is practised is unknown. Whilst this and other national guidelines on nutrition have been issued[2] there has as yet been no national review of the use of PN or its complications, and there exists little consensus opinion, at the clinical coalface, on its indications for use or administration. With this in mind the aim of this study was to look at the assessment, administration, catheter care and monitoring of patients nationally receiving PN.

1 – Method and data returns

Study aim

The primary aim of this study was to examine the process of care of patients receiving parenteral nutrition (PN) in hospital in order to identify remediable factors in the care received by these patients.

Objectives

The expert group identified six main thematic areas that would address the overall aim of the study and these will be addressed throughout the following chapters:

- Indication for PN
- Type of PN
- Prescribing PN
- Catheter choice, insertion and care
- Complications
- Nutrition teams

Hospital participation

National Health Service hospitals in England, Wales and Northern Ireland were expected to participate, as well as hospitals in the independent sector and public hospitals in the Isle of Man, Guernsey and Jersey.

Within each hospital, a named contact, referred to as the NCEPOD Local Reporter, acted as a link between NCEPOD and the hospital staff, facilitating case identification, dissemination of questionnaires and data collation.

Expert group

A multidisciplinary group of experts comprising consultants from gastroenterology, neonatology, paediatrics; nutrition nurse specialists, a dietitian, a pharmacist, a lay representative and a scientific advisor contributed to the design of the study and reviewed the findings.

Study population

Patients of all ages were eligible for inclusion if they received PN as an inpatient between 1st January 2008 and 31st March 2008 inclusive.

Exclusion criteria
The following patient groups were excluded:

- Patients receiving home parenteral nutrition when admitted

Case ascertainment

Patients receiving PN were identified retrospectively via pharmacies. Local Reporters then combined the patient information with details of the discharging clinician and sent this to NCEPOD in a password protected spreadsheet. These data were then imported into a secure database and subsequently up to two patients per consultant were selected at random and included in the study.

Questionnaires and case notes

There were two questionnaires used to collect data for this study, one clinician questionnaire per patient and one organisational questionnaire per hospital.

Clinician questionnaire

This questionnaire was sent to the consultant caring for the patient at the time of discharge. It may have been completed by that consultant or forwarded to a more appropriate member of the team who cared for the patient or had responsibility for the PN care. Information was requested on the indication for PN, patient assessment, PN prescription, venous access and catheter care, metabolic and non metabolic complications.

Organisational questionnaire

This questionnaire collected data on the prescription, manufacture and supply of PN. It also addressed the policies and protocols for each participating hospital with regard to PN and catheter care. Information was collected at the hospital level as it provided a better indication of the facilities available for a patient at the location where they were receiving care.

The organisational questionnaire was sent to the Medical Director or NCEPOD Local Reporter for completion in collaboration with relevant specialty input. Clinician questionnaires were either sent to the NCEPOD Local Reporter for dissemination or directly to the clinician involved. However, whichever method was used, it was requested that the completed questionnaires were returned directly to NCEPOD to maintain confidentiality.

Case notes

For each case to be peer reviewed, photocopies of the following case note extracts were requested:

- Clinical notes
- Nursing notes
- Nutrition notes
- Biochemistry results (LFT, U&E)
- Haematology results (e.g. FBC)
- Fluid balance charts (including urine output)
- Drug charts (including PN prescription chart)
- Nutritional charts
- Observation charts (including TPR, CVP)
- Weight chart
- Urinalysis
- X-ray/CT/ultrasound results
- Any operating notes

Advisor group

A multidisciplinary group of Advisors was recruited to review the case notes and associated questionnaires. The group of Advisors comprised clinicians from the following specialties: gastroenterology, paediatric gastroenterology, paediatric hepatology, intensive care medicine, general surgery, neonatology, paediatrics, clinical biochemistry and metabolic medicine, chemical pathology, dietitians, nutrition nurse specialists and pharmacists.

All questionnaires and case notes were anonymised by the non-clinical staff at NCEPOD. All patient, clinician and hospital identifiers were removed. Neither clinical co-ordinators at NCEPOD, nor the Advisors had access to any identifiable information.

After being anonymised each case was reviewed by one Advisor within a multidisciplinary group. At regular intervals throughout the meeting, the chair allowed a period of discussion for each Advisor to summarise their cases and ask for opinions from other specialties or raise aspects of a case for discussion.

The grading system below was used by the Advisors to grade the overall PN care each patient received.

Good practice: A standard that you would accept from yourself, your trainees and your institution.
Room for improvement: Aspects of *clinical* care that could have been better.
Room for improvement: Aspects of *organisational* care that could have been better.
Room for improvement: Aspects of both *clinical and organisational* care that could have been better.
Less than satisfactory: Several aspects of clinical and/or organisational care that were well below that you would accept from yourself, your trainees and your institution.
Insufficient information submitted to NCEPOD to assess the quality of care.

Quality and confidentiality

Each case was given a unique NCEPOD number so that cases could not easily be linked to a hospital.

The data from all questionnaires received were electronically scanned into a preset database. Prior to any analysis taking place, the data were cleaned to ensure that there were no duplicate records and that erroneous data had not been entered during scanning. Any fields that contained spurious data that could not be validated were removed.

Data analysis

Following cleaning of the quantitative data, descriptive data summaries were produced.

The qualitative data collected from the Advisors' opinions and free text answers in the clinician questionnaires were coded, where applicable, according to content to allow quantitative analysis. The data were reviewed by NCEPOD Clinical Co-ordinators and Clinical Researcher to identify the nature and frequency of recurring themes.

Case studies have been used at the end of this report to illustrate particular themes.

All data were analysed using Microsoft Access and Excel by the research staff at NCEPOD.

The findings of the report were reviewed by the Expert Group, Advisors and the NCEPOD Steering Group prior to publication.

Data returns

It can be seen from Figure 1.1 that 5527 patients from 218 hospitals were identified as meeting the inclusion criteria for the study. The study sample reduced to 3305 when the number of patients per consultant was limited to two and those patients where a PN prescription was written but not commenced, excluded. For a further 167 cases, NCEPOD was notified that the questionnaire could not be completed. Reasons for this included the case notes being lost and that the consultant was wrongly identified or had left the Trust. For the remaining 3138 included patients, a clinician questionnaire and/or case notes was received for 1948 cases (62%).

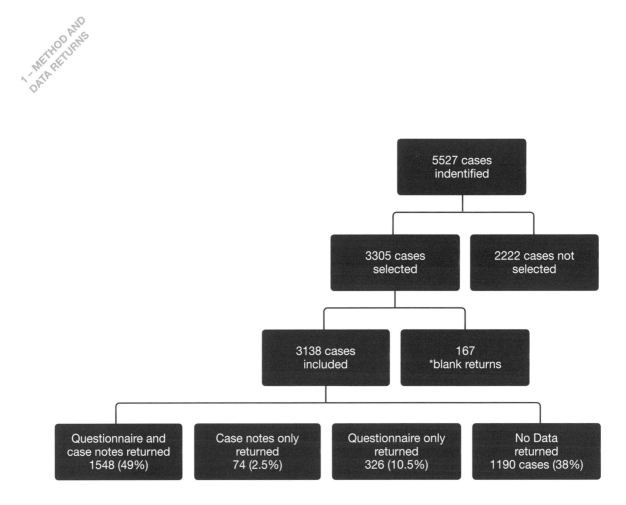

Figure 1.1 Data returns

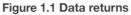

* *Blank returns were those cases where NCEPOD were informed that the relevant
   case notes could not be found or the consultant in charge of the patient at the
   time of their discharge had left the Trust.*

Study sample denominator data by chapter

Within this study the denominator will change for each
chapter and occasionally within each chapter. This is
because data has been taken from different sources
depending on the analysis required. For example in some
cases the data presented will be a total from a question
taken from the clinician questionnaire only, whereas some
analysis may have required the clinician questionnaire

and the Advisors' view taken from the case notes.
In total 877 adult, 70 paediatric and 264 neonatal cases
were assessed by the Advisors. The remainder of the
returned case note extracts were either too incomplete
for assessment or were returned after the final deadline
and last Advisor meeting. The number of clinician
questionnaires included in the analysis for each age
group was 1332 adults, 248 neonates and 66 paediatric
cases.

2 – Adult Parenteral Nutrition

Introduction

In this section we will look at the issues surrounding the prescription and administration of PN to adults. The decision to give PN is not one that should be taken lightly. Whilst PN is of undoubted value to those with a failing or inaccessible gut it does carry with it the risk of complications both related to the PN per se and the metabolic complications associated with the correction of nutritional/electrolyte deficiencies. There are also complications associated with the central venous catheter that the PN is delivered through (see Chapter 4). Thus when PN is being considered it is of great importance that an appropriate assessment of the patient has taken place and that following commencement of PN there are regular clinical reviews and monitoring. This is particularly important as this is a group of very sick patients with a high overall mortality from their underlying disease and it is vital that iatrogenic complications be avoided.

Adult Demographics

There were 877 patients in the adult group that were peer reviewed by the Advisors. The age range was 19-95, the average age being 65 and 544/877 (62%) were male. Figure 2.1 illustrates the age distribution in the adult group.

Overall care

From Table 2.1and Figure 2.2 it can be seen that the Advisors judged that 171/877 (19%) adult patients had PN care that was considered to represent good practice. Where it was found that there was room for improvement, this predominantly was in clinical care – 295/877 (34%). It was also identified that 209/877 (24%) of patients' PN care was judged deficient in terms of both clinical and organisational factors. In the opinion of the Advisors, care was considered less than satisfactory in 83/877 (9%) of cases.

Number of Patients

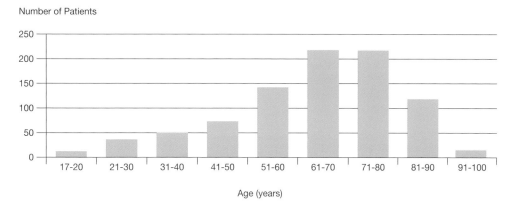

Age (years)

Figure 2.1 Age distribution of the adult study population

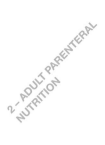

Table 2.1 Overall of assessment of PN care – Advisors' opinion

Overall Assessment	Number of patients	%
Good practice	171	19.5
Room for improvement – clinical	295	33.6
Room for improvement - organisational	81	9.2
Room for improvement - clinical and organisational	209	23.8
Less than satisfactory	83	9.5
Insufficient data	38	4.3
Total	877	

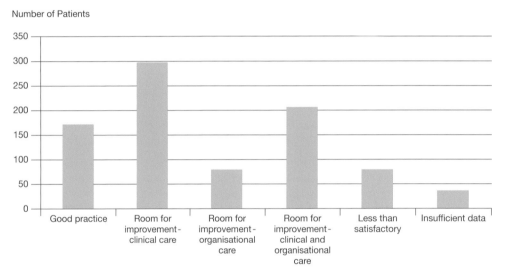

Figure 2.2 Overall of assessment of PN care – Advisors' opinion

These data present an issue of concern. An overall good standard of PN practice was found to be low in this group of patients who had intestinal failure. The remainder of the report will endeavour to establish the various factors involved in this finding. Nevertheless if this standard of care was uncovered in a group of patients with an alternative organ failure then these findings would be wholly unacceptable. NCEPOD recognises that such a sick group of patients warrants better care than that demonstrated here.

The specialties that the patients were under at the time the PN was administered are shown in Table 2.2, the indications for PN in Table 2.3 and the clinical areas the patients were in at the time of administration in Figure 2.3.

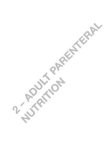

Table 2.2 Specialty under which PN was administered (clinician questionnaire)

Specialty	Number of patients	%
General surgery	294	22.1
Critical/Intensive care medicine	263	19.7
Colorectal surgery	238	17.9
Gastroenterology	94	7.1
Upper gastrointestinal surgery	74	5.6
Hepatology and pancreatic surgery	52	3.9
General medicine	29	2.2
Urology	28	2.1
Vascular surgery	28	2.1
Nephrology	19	1.4
Clinical haematology	18	1.4
Clinical oncology	16	1.2
Medical oncology	15	1.1
Gynaecology	15	1.1
Geriatric surgery	14	1.1
Trauma orthopaedics	11	< 1
Respiratory medicine	11	< 1
Cardiac surgery	11	< 1
Cardiothoracic surgery	11	< 1
Ear nose and throat	7	< 1
Breast surgery	6	< 1
Other	78	5.9
Total	**1332**	

Table 2.3 Documented indication for PN (answers may be multiple)

Documented indication for PN	Number of patients
Post-operative ileus	195
Post-surgical complications	124
Obstruction	119
Non functioning gut	109
Failure of enteric nutrition	109
Perforated/leaking gut	91
Other	86
No indication documented	73
Fistulae	48
No access for enteral nutrition	45
Cancer	30
Dysphagia	25
Malabsorption	23
Short bowel	22
Dysmotility	22
Infection	20
Crohn's disease	15
Pre-operative nutrition	14
Radiation enteritis	6
Chemotherapy	6
Radiation damage	5
Graft-Versus-Host disease	4
Volvulus	1

As can be seen the majority of patients within this study receiving PN were either gastrointestinal surgery, general surgery and/or critical care patients (Table 2.2). This reflects both complex surgical problems and multiple co-morbidities which require nutritional support. As such, a large number of patients in this study were given PN in a Level 3 setting which reflects both patient groups.

However, the majority of PN was given in the Level 1 setting (Figure 2.3). This reflects those patients who are not critically ill but require nutritional support for an ongoing disease process. It is entirely appropriate for PN to be given in a Level 1 setting providing there is a sufficient number of adequately PN-trained support staff available.

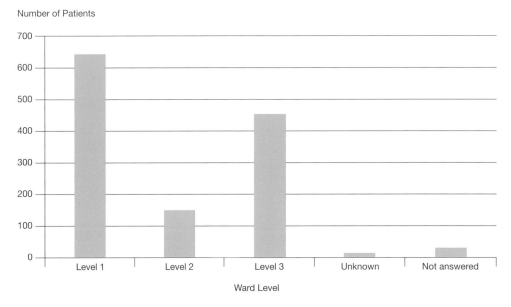

Number of Patients

Figure 2.3 Ward level under which PN was administered (clinician questionnaire)

The vast majority of PN was initiated during weekdays (707/846; 84% of cases; Table 2.4) and the time of day it was started was deemed appropriate in 79% (341/430) of cases where it was recorded (Figure 2.4). This is heartening as PN is not an emergency intervention in adults and there is rarely an indication for it to be started out of hours or at the weekend. This is because good

nutritional management requires forward thinking and timely assessment of nutritional needs. When the data were analysed to look at advisor opinion on inappropriate timing of initial PN versus day of the week, it can seen that where the Advisors judged timing to be inappropriate this tended to be more so at the weekend (Figure 2.4).

Table 2.4 Day of the week on which PN was commenced

Day PN was commenced	Number of patients	%
Monday	124	14.7
Tuesday	112	13.2
Wednesday	132	15.6
Thursday	141	16.7
Friday	198	23.4
Saturday	86	10.2
Sunday	53	6.3
Subtotal	846	
Unknown	31	
Total	877	

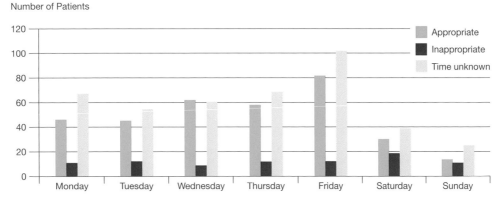

Number of Patients

Figure 2.4 Day of the week on which PN was administered and the Advisors' opinion on the appropriateness of the time of day it was commenced

Decision making

The responding clinicians were asked who made the decision to commence PN (Table 2.5) - the commonest response being a doctor (632/1279) or a combination of a doctor and dietitian (282/1279); approximately half the time they were a member of a nutrition team (Table 2.6). Whilst it is not unreasonable for the requirement for PN to be decided by a member of staff who is not part of a nutrition team it is desirable that a multidisciplinary nutrition team should have some input into the decision making process or, as a very minimum, be aware of the patient so as to ensure high standards of management and adequate monitoring.

Table 2.5 Designation of the person responsible for commencing PN

Designation	Number of patients
Doctor	632
Doctor/Dietitian	282
Doctor/Dietitian/Nurse	70
Doctor/Dietitian/Pharmacist/Nurse	59
Doctor/Other	18
Doctor/Pharmacist	12
Doctor/Dietitian/Other	9
Dietitian	53
Dietitian/Pharmacist/Doctor	49
Dietitian/Pharmacist	6
Nurse/Doctor	28
Nurse/Dietitian	17
Nurse/Dietitian/Pharmacist	15
Nurse	4
Pharmacist	6
Other	19
Subtotal	**1279**
Unknown	36
Not answered	17
Total	**1332**

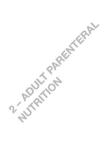

Table 2.6 Nutrition team involvement in the decision to commence PN

Nutrition team involved	Number of patients	%
Yes	610	52.7
No	547	47.3
Subtotal	**1157**	
Unknown	128	
Not answered	47	
Total	**1332**	

The clinicians completing the questionnaires stated that 690/1332 (52%) of patients had had a period of enteral feeding prior to the decision to commence PN. Table 2.7 shows the type of enteral feeding administered. As can be seen for the majority this enteral feeding was either oral supplements (sip feeds) or nasogastric feeding. It is perhaps a peculiar finding that so many patients went directly from oral supplements to parenteral nutrition without further utilisation of their gut through nasogastric or nasojejunal feeding. However in the absence of detailed data around specific disease processes in this group it may be unsafe to criticise this practice.

Table 2.7 Type of enteral feeding received prior to PN

Enteral feeding type	Number of patients
Oral supplements	272
Nasogastric	246
Oral supplement and nasogastric	57
Nasojejunal	30
Surgical jejunostomy	15
Percutaneous endoscopic gastrostomy	12
Oral supplement and nasojejunal	8
Nasogastric and nasojejunal	5
Oral supplement, nasogastric and nasojejunal	3
Nasogastric and percutaneous endoscopic gastrostomy	3
Distal Feeding	3
Percutaneous endoscopic gastrostomy –J	3
Radiologically inserted gastrostomy	2
Oral supplement and percutaneous endoscopic gastrostomy	1
Type of enteral feeding not defined	30
Subtotal	**690**
No enteral feeding	642
Total	**1332**

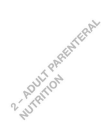

For those patients who had not had any enteral feeding prior to PN the mean number of days without nutritional support was 7.5 and the mode 2 (range 0-90 days). According to the clinicians completing the questionnaires the mean number of days between the decision to start PN and its commencement was 1 day (0-17 days).

In the opinion of the Advisors there was an unreasonable delay in the recognition of the need for PN in 16% (128/798) of patients and a delay in starting PN in 9% (71/782) (Tables 2.8 and 2.9). Whilst this number is small there should never be an unreasonable delay between the decision to start PN and its administration. It may be arguable that an adult patient is unlikely to come to harm from delays in administration of PN, but it is equally as arguable that the management of any serious medical condition should not be hampered by delays of any kind. A delay in medical treatment represents poor organisation and/or communication thus it is undesirable, unnecessary and remediable.

Table 2.8 Delay in recognition of PN requirement

Unreasonable delay in recognising the need for PN	Number of patients	%
Yes	128	16.0
No	670	84.0
Subtotal	**798**	
Unknown/insufficient data	79	
Total	**877**	

Table 2.9 Delay in commencing PN once the need was recognised

Unreasonable delay in starting PN	Number of patients	%
Yes	71	9.1
No	711	90.9
Subtotal	**782**	
Unknown/insufficient data	95	
Total	**877**	

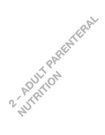

Number of Patients

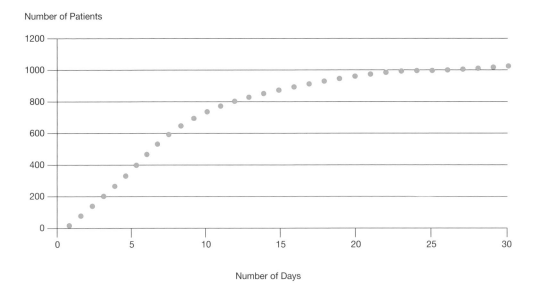

Number of Days

Figure 2.5 Number of days for which the patient received PN (clinician questionnaire)

The average duration of PN was 12.2 days, with a range of 1-276 days, the median being eight days. Figure 2.5 shows the data for those patients who received PN for 30 days or less (1053/1132 patients). Seventy nine patients received PN for more than 30 days, this question was not answered for 200 patients.

It is of concern that 177 patients had PN for three days or less. This may reflect bad decision making with respect to the necessity for PN or possibly that problems, such as post-operative ileus, resolved more quickly than expected in these patients.

In summary these data show that nutrition teams were under utilised in the decision to start PN, and there were palpable delays for some patients in the administration of PN once the decision to start it has been made; in addition PN is being given for very short intervals in some cases. In view of the expense of providing PN and its potential for complications, decision making around its prescription needs to be robust, in terms of clinical necessity, promptness of delivery and predicted duration.

Prescription

There are three main types of PN. Multi-chamber 'off-the-shelf' bags (these require the addition of vitamins and trace elements), multi-chamber bags with other additives (usually additional electrolytes), and individually compounded 'bespoke' bags. NICE have clearly stated that all multi-chamber bags should have vitamins added prior to administration.[2]

The type of PN prescribed is shown in Table 2.10. The commonest prescription was found to be multi-chamber bags and accounted for 43% of cases (399/935). Multi-chamber bags with micronutrient additives made up 13% (124/935), with multi-chamber bags with micronutrient and tailored additions making up 22% (208/935). The prevalence of named-patient individually compounded or 'bespoke' bags was relatively lower at 22% (204/935). This distribution represents the likelihood that most patients were started on stocked pre-compounded bags (so-called starter bags) with only a few patients requiring specifically compounded 'bespoke' bags at the outset, or other types of bag were simply not readily available.

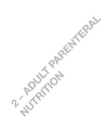

These data also suggest that a large proportion of patients were being given pre-compounded bags without micronutrient supplements which would be dangerous practice and go against NICE guidelines. However, it is possible that this figure represents a failure of the responding clinicians to answer the question correctly - although the figure is somewhat high for this explanation, and the multiple choice question gave all possible compositions of PN as answer options. Additionally, there was anecdotal evidence from the Expert Group that such poor practice is indeed highly prevalent in hospitals. Thus if this figure is truly representative it shows a very poor standard of initial PN prescription which goes against current NICE guidelines.

Table 2.10 First type of PN given

Type of PN	Number of patients	%
Off the shelf	399	42.7
Off the shelf and micronutrients	124	13.3
Off the shelf and micronutrients and tailored additions	208	22.2
Bespoke	204	21.8
Subtotal	**935**	
Unknown	328	
Not answered	69	
Total	**1332**	

The nutritional requirements of the patient were most commonly determined by a dietitian alone in 509/1332 (38%) of cases with the next commonest assessors being a dietitian and a doctor 142/1332 (11%). Regardless of who determined the nutritional requirements they were part of a nutrition team 80% of the time (931/1166; Table 2.11).

Table 2.11 Nutrition team involvement in determining the patient's PN nutritional requirements

Nutrition team involved	Number of patients	%
Yes	931	79.8
No	235	20.2
Subtotal	1166	
Unknown	**128**	
Not answered	38	
Total	**1332**	

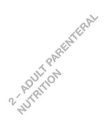

Table 2.12 Advisors' opinion on the appropriateness of the first PN prescription

First PN appropriate for the patient	Number of patients	%
Yes	425	85.0
No	75	15.0
Subtotal	500	
Unknown/insufficient data	377	
Total	877	

The PN prescription was most commonly signed by a doctor 789/1076 (73%); however only 40% of prescribers were part of a nutrition team. It should be noted that according to the clinicians completing the questionnaires there were 256 cases where the identity of the prescriber was not known. This indicates poor documentation.

According to the Advisors 75/500 (15%) of first PN prescriptions in this study were inappropriate (Table 2.12).

As stated earlier it is important that a multidisciplinary nutrition team is involved in patient care to some degree and these data show that in some cases there was an absence of their involvement in initial decision making, assessment of nutritional requirements and prescription.

Indications

The Advisors deemed that in just over a quarter of patients in this study (232/808) the PN was administered for an inappropriate indication (Table 2.13). PN should only be given where there is a clear and valid indication as its administration is associated with the possibility of complications, some of which may be life-threatening.

Furthermore, the Advisors judged that for the 73 patients where no indication for PN was documented (see Table 2.3), the use of PN was inappropriate for 50/55 patients (for 18 patients no judgment could be made).

Table 2.13 Advisors' opinion on whether PN was indicated

Appropriate indication for PN	Number of patients	%
Yes	576	71.3
No	232	28.7
Subtotal	808	
Insufficient data	69	
Total	877	

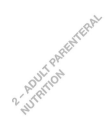

Of the 232 patients where the Advisors felt that PN was not indicated, data on the total duration of PN was available for 195 patients. The average length of time PN was given to this group of patients was 7.6 days. These data, combined with Figure 2.5 give rise to the suspicion that patients may be being given PN for inappropriately short lengths of time; this being further compounded by the opinion of the Advisors that some of these patients did not require PN at all. This exposes patients to unnecessary risks and represents a serious resource issue as PN is an expensive commodity.

Additionally, in a third (271/829) of the study patients there was judged to be inadequate consideration of enteral feeding (Table 2.14). When making the decision to give PN the possibility of giving enteral nutrition needs to be actively excluded. The exclusion should be based either on the inaccessibility of the gut or the extent of the intestinal failure. In some circumstances both enteral and parenteral nutrition are indicated. If PN is the appropriate nutritional support then that should be recognised quickly and started without delay. This does not mean that adult PN should be started out of hours or at weekends.

Table 2.14 Advisors' opinion on whether there was adequate consideration of enteral nutrition

Adequate consideration given	Number of patients	%
Yes	558	67.3
No	271	32.7
Subtotal	829	
Insufficient data	48	
Total	877	

Clinical Assessment, Monitoring and Complications

It is of the utmost importance that before the delivery of PN there should be an adequate assessment of the nutritional requirements of the patient both in terms of their total energy requirement and biochemical status. For more than half (399/738) of the study patients this assessment was found by the Advisors to be inadequate (Table 2.15).

Table 2.15 Advisors' opinion on whether the patient received an adequate biochemical and nutritional assessment prior to the commencement of PN

Adequate assessment given	Number of patients	%
Yes	339	45.9
No	399	54.1
Subtotal	738	
Unknown/insufficient data	139	
Total	877	

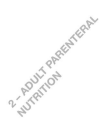

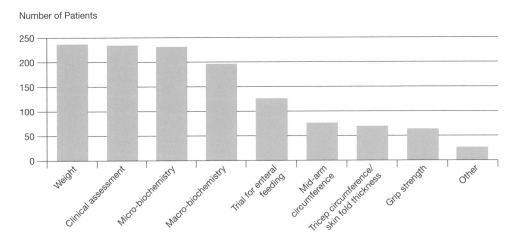

Number of Patients

Deficiencies in Assessment

Figure 2.6 Deficiencies in biochemical and nutritional assessment (answers may be multiple)

The most common omissions were an adequate clinical assessment, micro- and macro-biochemical review and omission of weight (Figure 2.6). This is a surprising finding as it is difficult to understand how the need for PN can be established unless the patient has, as a minimum, had a baseline clinical assessment and measurement of weight. However, these basic parameters were apparently omitted in a number of patients.

As with all clinical parameters, nutritional requirements should be clearly documented in the case notes. For half of all patients (448/856) there was no evidence of their nutritional requirements being documented (Table 2.16).

Once nutritional requirements have been established there should also be a treatment goal documented, so that all staff and the patient understand the purpose and endpoint of the PN. The Advisors found no evidence of a treatment goal being documented in 398/845 (47%) patients.

As PN is a metabolically active substance its administration is unsafe unless there is regular clinical and biochemical monitoring. Following the administration of PN the Advisors found that there was inadequate monitoring of the patient in 43.3% (296/683) patients (Table 2.17).

Table 2.16 Documentation of patients' nutritional requirements

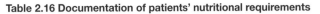

Requirements documented	Number of patients	%
Yes	408	47.7
No	448	52.3
Subtotal	**856**	
Insufficient data	21	
Total	**877**	

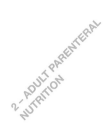

Table 2.17 Advisors' opinion on the adequacy of clinical and biochemical monitoring

Adequate monitoring	Number of patients	%
Yes	387	56.7
No	296	43.3
Subtotal	683	
Unknown/insufficient data	194	
Total	877	

The major monitoring deficiencies are shown in Figure 2.7.

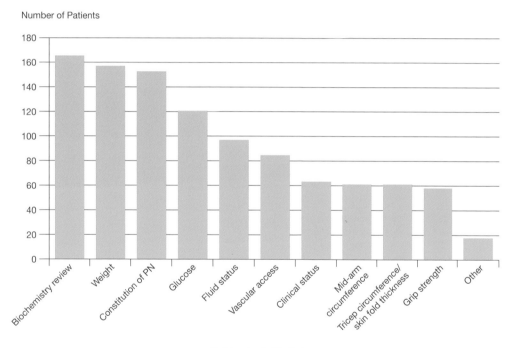

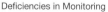

Figure 2.7 Deficiencies in monitoring (answers may be multiple)

It is of considerable concern to see that basic monitoring modalities such as weight and biochemical review were being omitted. It seems improbable that PN can be safely administered if biochemistry is not being monitored nor can endpoints be established if weight is not being measured. A failure to measure weight may be acceptable in some patients owing to a lack of mobility – such as those on Level 3. In addition, Level 3 patients may have rapid shifts in fluid balance making some weights spurious, however to a large extent this also applies to all patients with intestinal failure and in itself should not be used as an excuse not to attempt to measure weight or anthropometric response.

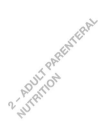

Once PN was established, the Advisors judged that there was an adequate frequency of reviews (785/818), including the number of senior clinical reviews (631/688), for the majority of patients. Despite this, the Advisors found evidence that 249/634 (39.3%) patients developed metabolic complications whilst being given PN (Table 2.18). The commonest of these were hypophosphataemia and hypokalaemia (Figure 2.8). Even with good clinical management not all biochemical disturbances can necessarily be eliminated; however the high prevalence of hypophosphataemia is surprising considering this is readily recognised as an essential biochemical marker to monitor, and can be an early indicator of re-feeding syndrome.

Where data were available the Advisors found that 81/164 (49.4%) of these metabolic complications were avoidable (Table 2.19) with 30/194 (15.5%) managed inappropriately once recognised (Table 2.20). It is not unreasonable to surmise that if monitoring had been adequate then many of these complications may have been avoided. As such it is paradoxical that despite evidence of adequate senior reviews monitoring was deficient and complications rife. This suggests that those undertaking the reviews may have had either insufficient experience to allow them to be aware of and recognise complications, or more controversially, may have simply exhibited a generally poor standard of clinical care.

Table 2.18 Evidence of metabolic complications

Metabolic complications	Number of patients	%
Yes	249	39.3
No	385	60.7
Subtotal	**634**	
Insufficient data	243	
Total	**877**	

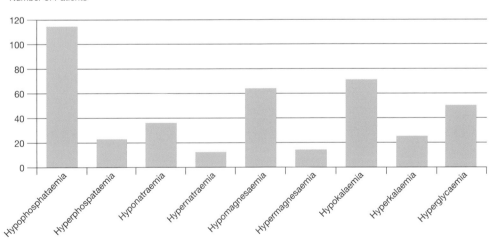

Number of Patients

Metabolic Complications

Figure 2.8 Types of metabolic complications (answers may be multiple)

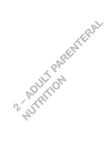

Intravenous Fluids

There is a perception that junior medical staff can often overlook the fact that PN being a fluid provides a significant load to the circulation over the period of administration. This oversight can lead to additional intravenous fluids being administered. In some circumstances this may be appropriate but in others this will be unnecessary and may lead to peripheral and pulmonary oedema as well as sodium overload. The Advisors found that 513/681 (75.3%) patients had been given additional IV fluids of which 63/334 (18.9%)

were of an inappropriate type (e.g. crystalloid/colloid) and 93/329 (28.3%) were an inappropriate volume (Tables 2.21 – 2.23). Thus the perception that extraneous and unnecessary IV fluids are being administered to patients on PN is borne out by these data. Based on this finding NCEPOD would support greater education amongst junior doctors around the administration of intravenous fluids, through the widespread distribution of the *'Guidelines on Intravenous Fluid Therapy for Adult Surgical Patients'* (GIFTASUP)[3], and its co-administration with PN in particular.

Table 2.19 Advisors' opinion on whether the metabolic complications that developed were avoidable

Avoidable metabolic complications	Number of patients	%
Yes	81	49.4
No	83	50.6
Subtotal	164	
Unknown/insufficient data	85	
Total	249	

Table 2.20 Advisors' opinion on whether the metabolic complications that developed were managed appropriately

Appropriately managed	Number of patients	%
Yes	164	84.5
No	30	15.5
Subtotal	194	
Unknown/insufficient data	55	
Total	249	

Table 2.21 Evidence of additional IV fluids

Fluids given	Number of patients	%
Yes	513	75.3
No	168	24.7
Subtotal	681	
Insufficient data	196	
Total	877	

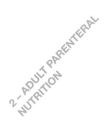

Table 2.22 Advisors' opinion on the appropriateness of the type of additional fluid

Appropriate fluids	Number of patients	%
Yes	271	81.1
No	63	18.9
Subtotal	334	
Insufficient data	179	
Total	513	

Table 2.23 Advisors' opinion on the appropriateness of the volume of additional fluid

Volume appropriate	Number of patients	%
Yes	236	71.7
No	93	28.3
Subtotal	329	
Insufficient data	184	
Total	513	

Re-feeding Syndrome

Re-feeding syndrome (RFS) is the occurrence of circulatory overload with potentially fatal cardio-respiratory failure on commencement of nutritional therapy following a period of starvation. It occurs due to the movement of sodium out of, and phosphate and magnesium into cells as a physiological response to re-feeding. The chance of it developing can be reduced by the recognition that the patient is at risk, the administration of prophylactic vitamins and intravenous phosphate, as well as the avoidance of sodium and water overload. Further risk reduction can be achieved by initiating PN at slow infusion rates before gradually building up caloric intake.

Data from earlier in this report illustrated that hypophosphataemia was common (Figure 2.8); however it should be noted that amongst the Advisors there was consensus agreement that, for the purposes of this study, they would not define RFS as a drop in phosphate only. The following data should be interpreted with this in mind. In the opinion of the Advisors 455/755 (60.3%) of patients

were at risk of RFS (Table 2.24) but in only half these patients was such risk documented by the clinical team (Table 2.25). This raises the question as to whether RFS is simply not being considered as a possibility or whether it is being considered but the risk not quantified and documented. Re-feeding syndrome is an important complication of feeding malnourished patients and further considers that this should be documented wherever it may pose a potential problem.

Of those patients where RFS was a documented risk the Advisors found that it actually occurred in 33/174 (19%) patients (Table 2.26). Furthermore it occurred in 20 patients despite adequate precautions being taken (Table 2.27). But perhaps more interestingly in the 28 patients who did not receive adequate precautions it occurred in only 13/28 (Table 2.27). Thus re-feeding syndrome when predicted may not always be avoided despite adequate precautions and when the risk is overlooked, it does not always occur. This perhaps suggests that the issues around re-feeding syndrome, especially with respect to its likelihood of occurrence, need to be robustly debated; especially with respect to the realistic risk of it actually occurring.

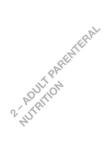

Table 2.24 Advisors' opinion on whether the patient was at risk of RFS

At risk	Number of patients	%
Yes	455	60.3
No	300	39.7
Subtotal	**755**	
Unknown/insufficient data	122	
Total	**877**	

Table 2.25 Risk of RFS documented in notes

Risk documented	Number of patients	%
Yes	224	49.8
No	226	50.2
Subtotal	**450**	
Insufficient data	5	
Total	**455**	

Table 2.26 Evidence that RFS occurred amongst those patients documented to be at risk occurred

Re-feeding syndrome occurred	Number of patients	%
Yes	33	19.0
No	141	81.0
Subtotal	**174**	
Insufficient data/unknown	50	
Total	**224**	

Table 2.27 Occurrence of RFS and the Advisors' opinion on adequacy of precautions

	Adequate precautions		
Re-feeding syndrome occurred	Yes	No	Total
Yes	20	13	**33**
No	126	15	**141**
Total	**146**	**28**	**174**

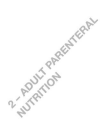

Key Findings

- Good practice around PN care was identified in only 19% (171/877) of patients in this study.
- Inadequate consideration was given to enteral nutrition in a third (271/829) of patients in the opinion of the Advisors.
- PN was administered for an inappropriate indication to 29% (232/808) of study patients.
- In the view of the Advisors there was an unreasonable delay in recognition of the need for PN in 16% (128/798) of patients.
- There was an unreasonable delay in starting PN once the need was recognised in 9% (71/782) of patients in this study.
- There were deficiencies in the assessment and monitoring of patients in 54% (399/738) of patients on PN.
- Metabolic complications occurred in 40% (249/634) of patients and in 49% (81/164) these were judged by the Advisors to be avoidable.
- Additional IV fluids were given to 75% (513/681) of patients and in 28% (93/329) of these cases this was judged to be of an inappropriate volume.
- There was poor documentation of nutritional issues.

Recommendations

- PN should only be given when enteral nutrition has been considered, and excluded, as either inappropriate and/or impracticable. However situations may arise where both enteral and parenteral nutrition are necessary. (Consultants)
- Where the possibility exists that a patient may require PN this should be recognised early. Subsequently, should PN become a clinical necessity, this should be rapidly actioned and PN started at the earliest opportunity. However, there is rarely, if ever, an indication to start adult PN out of normal working hours. (Consultants)
- Patient assessment should be robust to ensure that PN is the appropriate nutritional intervention and that adequate PN is administered. The clinical purpose and goal of the PN should be documented. (Consultants)
- Regular documented clinical monitoring, of the patient and PN prescription, should be mandatory. Monitoring should include daily weights (where possible) and documentation of the success of the PN within the overall clinical picture. (Consultants)
- Regular documented biochemical monitoring should be mandatory to ensure avoidable metabolic complications never occur. (Clinical Directors)
- Additional intravenous fluids should only be prescribed where there has been an active assessment of the volume of PN already being administered and there is clear indication that further fluids/electrolytes are required. (Consultants)
- There must be active under/post graduate education about the role of PN, its complications and side effects. (Deaneries)
- All hospitals should have a PN proforma which includes: Indication for PN; Treatment goal; Risk of and precautions taken against re-feeding syndrome; PN prescription; Weight and Biochemical monitoring. (Medical Directors)

3 – Neonatal Parenteral Nutrition

Introduction

Nutritional support for sick, term and preterm, neonates is essential to meet requirements for growth and neurobiological development. The nutritional requirements of these infants will vary depending on many factors. These include gestational age, birth weight, respiratory and cardiovascular function, acquired gut dysfunction such as necrotising enterocolitis (NEC) and congenital alimentary tract causes.

The goals of nutrition for the sick neonate are debated but an approximation to normal intra-uterine and postnatal growth would seem logical. The routes for feeding and the nutritional constituents should be matched to the requirements of each neonate [4-6].

Whilst commencing enteral feeding as early as possible following birth should be the primary aim, this is not always possible and either complete or partial supplementation with parenteral nutrition (PN) may be required until full enteral feeding can be established. The role of PN in the majority of preterm neonates is to bridge the gap of functional gut immaturity until enteral nutrition can be established.

Parenteral nutrition for neonates via a central venous catheter has been used for the last 40 years[7] but it is only in the last 20 years that it has been increasingly part of routine clinical practice within neonatal units. Evidence now exists that in extremely low birth weight (ELBW) neonates PN should be started soon after birth so that the full nutritional value can be achieved early in postnatal life[8-11]. Despite this evidence many neonatal units delay the introduction and rate of progression of amino acids and lipids in this group of neonates[12,13].

Guidelines on PN in infants and children have been published by the European Society of Paediatric Gastroenterology, Hepatology and Nutrition (ESPGHAN), the European Society for Clinical Nutrition and Metabolism (ESPEN) and the European Society of Paediatric Research (ESPR)[14]. These guidelines cover:

- Energy requirements
- Composition of PN
  - Amino acids, lipid, carbohydrate etc
  - Fluid and electrolyte balance
  - Additives
- Organisation of PN
- Nutrition teams
- Prescribing
- Monitoring
- Weaning

Administration of PN in neonates is complex, technically demanding and requires considerable skill and judgement. It is important to determine the correct nutritional and fluid requirements, provide adequate and appropriate PN constituents, obtain adequate vascular access, use suitable delivery techniques and undertake careful biochemical and clinical monitoring.

Devastating complications can occur from PN including component incompatibility, drug interactions, sepsis and metabolic derangement. Furthermore complications related to vascular access can occur (see Chapter 4).

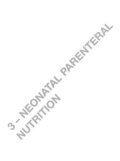

The best organisational model in the administration of PN on neonatal units has yet to be established. However to ensure safe delivery there should be good communication and team working amongst all those involved in the administration of PN including clinicians, pharmacists, dietitians and experts in nutrition[15,16]. Furthermore it is essential that those responsible for the care of the neonate who requires PN should have adequate education and training in these techniques[14].

In this study of 264 neonates from 74 hospitals, NCEPOD has undertaken the first case based peer review of PN in neonates across England, Wales, Northern Ireland and the Offshore Islands.

Neonatal Demographics

The gestational age of the 264 neonates included in this study is shown in Figure 3.1, 155 (59%) were of 30 weeks gestational age or less. This reflects the incidence of premature and low birth weight infants in England and Wales and highlights that immaturity of gastrointestinal function is one of the major indications for PN[17].

Overall quality of PN care

The Advisors who assessed the sample of neonates who received PN included in this study were asked to form an opinion on the overall quality of the PN care. The Advisors judged that only 62/264 (23.5%) of patients had PN care that was considered to represent good practice. It was considered that there was room for improvement in clinical care in 107/264 (40.5%), room for improvement in organisational care in 25/264 (9.5%) and room for improvement in both clinical and organisational care in 49/264 (18.6%). In the opinion of the Advisors, care was considered less than satisfactory in 12/264 (4.5%) of cases (Table 3.1 and Figure 3.2).

Number of Patients

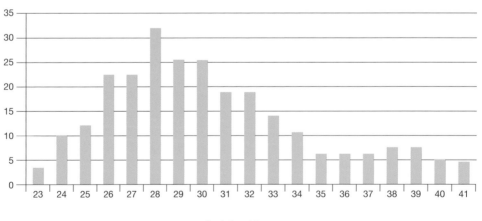

Gestational Age

Figure 3.1 Gestational age of neonatal study population

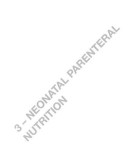

Table 3.1 Overall of assessment of PN care – Advisors' opinion

Overall Assessment	Number of patients	%
Good practice	62	23.5
Room for improvement – clinical	107	40.5
Room for improvement – organisational	25	9.5
Room for improvement – clinical and organisational	49	18.6
Less than satisfactory	12	4.5
Insufficient data	9	3.4
Total	**264**	

Number of Patients

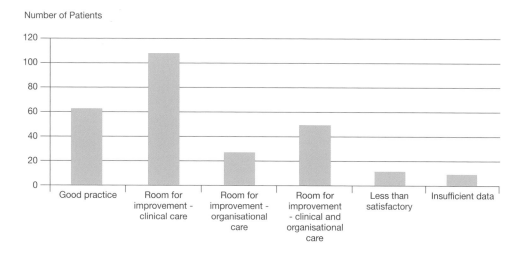

Figure 3.2 Overall of assessment of PN care – Advisors' opinion

The fact that the Advisors who undertook the peer review process found such a deficiency in the care of PN in neonates is not something that can be easily ignored. Parenteral nutrition is a fundamental therapeutic component of the care of the sick and premature neonate. The fact that the Advisors were of the opinion that in 193/264 (73%) cases this care was considered to be less than 'good practice' is explored further.

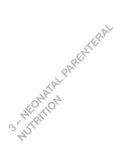

Table 3.2 Type of ward where PN was administered (clinician questionnaire)

Type of ward	Number of patients	%
Neonatal Unit	229	93.1
Paediatric Critical Care	14	5.7
Paediatric Medical	2	<1
Paediatric Surgical	1	<1
Subtotal	**246**	
Not answered	2	
Total	**248**	

Table 3.3 Level of ward on which PN was administered (clinician questionnaire)

Level of care	Number of patients	%
Level 3	177	76.6
Level 2	46	19.9
Level 1	8	3.5
Subtotal	**231**	
Not answered	15	
Unknown	2	
Total	**248**	

The majority of the neonates were cared for on Neonatal Units in a Level 3 or Level 2 environment (Tables 3.2 and 3.3)

There was a wide variety of indications for PN documented in the case notes (Table 3.4). The majority were for immaturity of gut function due to prematurity.

Decision making

In many circumstances enteral feeding should be the first choice for nutritional support and consequently careful consideration should be given before commencing PN.

The Advisors were asked for their opinion as to whether adequate consideration had been given to enteral feeding (Table 3.5). They deemed that this had not been the case in 23 neonates.

Furthermore, the Advisors judged that the indication for PN was inappropriate in 16 neonates (Table 3.6). Reasons that Advisors gave for inappropriate indications for PN included babies who were already established on enteral feeding or where enteral feeding would have been more suitable to meet the babies' requirements e.g. good size or late preterm babies. There were also two babies with severe birth asphyxia where treatment withdrawal may have been the best course.

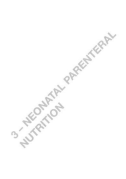

Table 3.4 Indications for PN (answers may be multiple)

Indication for PN	Number of patients
Immaturity of gut function	191
Necrotising enterocolitis	24
Congenital anomalies, gut	15
Non functioning gut	7
Dysmotility	5
Perforated/leaking gut	3
Congenital anomalies, non gut	2
Short bowel	2
Failure of enteral nutrition	2
Infection	2
Post operative ileus	2
Obstruction	1

Table 3.5 Advisors' opinion on whether there was adequate consideration of enteral nutrition

Adequate consideration given	Number of patients	%
Yes	228	90.8
No	23	9.2
Subtotal	251	
Insufficient data	13	
Total	264	

Table 3.6 Advisors' opinion on whether PN was indicated

Appropriate indication	Number of patients	%
Yes	244	93.8
No	16	6.2
Subtotal	260	
Insufficient data	4	
Total	264	

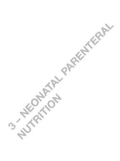

Even though in the majority of neonates the Advisors judged that the indication for PN was appropriate, in 71/252 (28.2%) of cases it was considered that there was an unreasonable delay in recognising the need for PN (Table 3.7). Many of these babies were extremely premature and of low birth weight and therefore with minimal nutritional reserve. Most of the delays were in the order of a few days from birth; however in some cases the delays were up to a week or more during which inadequate nutritional support had been given.

Due to the skilled judgement required in deciding to commence PN one would expect that this would be undertaken at senior level in conjunction with other members of the nutritional support team. The clinicians completing the patient care questionnaire were asked about the personnel, medical specialty and grade involved in these decisions (Tables 3.8-3.10). It can be seen that the majority of these decisions were made by consultants in neonatology.

Table 3.7 Delay in recognition of PN requirement – Advisors' opinion

Unreasonable delay	Number of patients	%
Yes	71	28.2
No	181	71.8
Subtotal	**252**	
Unknown/insufficient data	12	
Total	**264**	

Table 3.8 Designation of the person responsible for making the decision to commence PN (clinician questionnaire)

Designation	Number of patients
Doctor	216
Doctor/Pharmacist	6
Doctor/Nurse	4
Doctor/Dietitian/Pharmacist	3
Doctor/Dietitian	2
Doctor/Nurse/Dietitian	1
Doctor/Other	5
Doctor/Dietitian/Pharmacist/Nurse	1
Subtotal	**238**
Unknown	7
Not answered	3
Total	**248**

Once the decision to commence PN has been made there should not be any unreasonable delay before its commencement. The clinicians completing the patient care questionnaire were asked for the time interval between the decision to start PN and its commencement (Table 3.11). While in 211 neonates PN was started within a day of this decision, in 14 cases there was a delay of two days or more. Reasons for these delays included PN not being available at the weekend (3 patients), difficult intravenous access (2 patients) and awaiting stabilisation of the patient (2 patients).

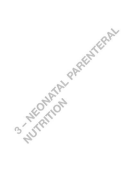

Table 3.9 Specialty of doctor making the decision to commence PN (clinician questionnaire)

Specialty of doctor	Number of patients	%
Neonatology	157	70.4
Paediatrics	37	16.6
Paediatric surgery	18	8.1
Paediatric ICU	4	1.8
Other	7	3.1
Subtotal	**223**	
Not answered/Doctor not involved	25	
Total	**248**	

Table 3.10 Grade of doctor making the decision to commence PN (clinician questionnaire)

Grade of doctor	Number of patients	%
Consultant	187	88.6
ST3 or above*	19	9.0
SAS	3	1.4
Other	2	<1
Subtotal	**211**	
Not answered/doctor not involved	37	
Total	**248**	

* For the purpose of these data ST3 was equivalent to SpR3

Table 3.11 Time between decision to start PN and its commencement (clinician questionnaire)

Time (days)	Number of patients	%
0	162	72.0
1	49	21.8
2	10	4.4
3	1	<1
5	2	<1
10	1	<1
Subtotal	**225**	
Not answered	23	
Total	**248**	

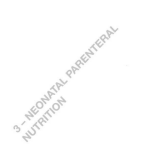

The Advisors were asked if they considered there to be an unreasonable delay between the decision to start PN and its commencement (Table 3.12). In 36/210 (17.1%) cases they were of this view. These were nearly all in extremely premature or extremely low birth weight babies.

It is possible that delays occurred because of the decision to start PN occurring at a time of day when constituting PN may not be possible. However in this study the majority of decisions to start PN occurred during normal working hours (196/233) so this is unlikely to be the cause of these delays.

Assessments

Before the initiation of PN a thorough nutritional assessment should be undertaken[14]. This should include:
- Medical history
- Physical examination including weight, head circumference
- Full blood count (including platelets and differential white count)
- Glucose, electrolytes, urea, creatinine
- Calcium, phosphate
- Albumin, liver function tests

Table 3.12 Delay in commencing PN once the need was recognised - Advisors' opinion

Unreasonable delay	Number of patients	%
Yes	36	17.1
No	174	82.9
Subtotal	210	
Unknown/insufficient data	54	
Total	264	

Table 3.13 Advisors' opinion on whether the patient received an adequate biochemical and nutritional assessment prior to the commencement of PN

Adequate assessment	Number of patients	%
Yes	194	90.2
No	21	9.8
Subtotal	215	
Unknown/insufficient data	49	
Total	264	

The Advisors were asked to give their opinion on the adequacy of the nutritional assessment. While the majority of the assessments were deemed adequate, for 21/215 (9.8%) patients this was not the case (Table 3.13).

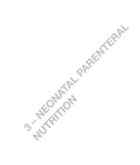

Number of Patients

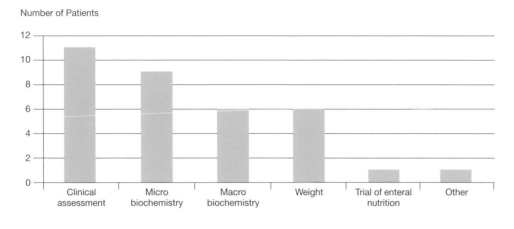

Deficiencies in Assessment

**Figure 3.3 Deficiencies in biochemical and nutritional assessment
(answers may be multiple)**

The Advisors were further asked to indicate where deficiencies in the assessment were found (Figure 3.3).

Having made a nutritional assessment, the individual requirements and goal for nutritional support should be determined. These should be documented clearly in the case notes. On review of the case notes the Advisors could only find evidence that these nutritional requirements had been documented in 70/250 (28%) of neonates (Table 3.14). Of these 70 cases there was inadequate detail of the requirements in 20 cases.

Table 3.14 Documentation of patient's nutritional requirements

Requirements documented	Number of patients	%
Yes	70	28.0
No	180	72.0
Subtotal	**250**	
Insufficient data	14	
Total	**264**	

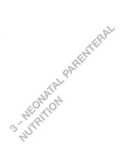
While at first sight these findings may be considered an indication of poor care it must be remembered that in many circumstances, particularly for preterm infants the requirements and nutritional goals would be considered self evident. However it would not be unreasonable for neonatal units to have an agreed policy for nutritional requirements plus a proforma that includes this information tailored for each infant that could be placed in the case notes. Interestingly, unlike the decision to initiate PN which is predominately undertaken by neonatal consultants (Table 3.15), the requirements were determined in 70/182 (38.5%) cases by non consultant grades (Table 3.16). Perhaps unsurprisingly this was more frequently undertaken in conjunction with pharmacists (Table 3.17).

Table 3.15 Specialty of doctor determining the patient's nutritional requirements (clinician questionnaire)

Specialty of doctor	Number of patients	%
Neonatology	137	70.3
Paediatrics	41	21.0
Paediatric surgery	5	2.6
Paediatric ICU	4	2.1
Other	8	4.1
Subtotal	**195**	
Not answered	53	
Total	**248**	

Table 3.16 Grade of doctor determining the patient's nutritional requirements (clinician questionnaire)

Grade of doctor	Number of patients	%
Consultant	112	61.5
ST3 or above*	57	31.3
ST2*	5	2.7
NCCG	3	1.6
SAS	3	1.6
FY	2	1.1
Subtotal	**182**	
Not answered	66	
Total	**248**	

* For the purpose of these data ST3 was equivalent to SpR3 and ST2 equivalent to SpR1-2

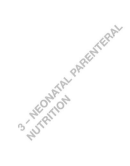

Table 3.17 Designation of the person responsible for determining the patients' PN nutritional requirements (clinician questionnaire)

Designation	Number of patients	%
Doctor	97	39.1
Doctor/Pharmacist	88	35.5
Pharmacist	16	6.5
Doctor/Pharmacist/Dietitian	11	4.4
Doctor/Pharmacist/Nurse	8	3.2
Doctor/Dietitian	5	2.0
Other	20	8.1
Unknown	3	1.2
Total	**248**	

Prescribing

Once the decision has been made to commence PN and the requirements have been determined, a clear prescription should be written. This should be done firstly to inform the pharmacy department of the composition of the PN and secondly to provide sufficient information to the nursing staff to deliver the PN safely.

Tables 3.18, 3.19 and 3.20 show that prescribing was mainly done by middle grade trainees. While this may be appropriate in most circumstances, one would wish to ensure that trainee doctors had adequate senior supervision when prescribing PN.

Table 3.18 Designation of the person that signed the prescription

Designation	Number of patients	%
Doctor	188	75.8
Doctor/Pharmacist	28	11.3
Pharmacist	16	6.5
Doctor/Pharmacist/Nurse	4	1.6
Other	8	3.2
Unknown	4	1.6
Total	**248**	

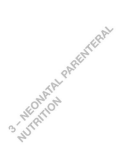

Table 3.19 Specialty of doctor signing the prescription

Specialty of doctor	Number of patients	%
Neonatology	140	71.4
Paediatrics	42	21.4
Paediatric surgery	4	2.0
Other	10	5.1
Subtotal	**196**	
Not applicable	25	
Not answered	27	
Total	**248**	

Table 3.20 Grade of doctor signing the prescription

Grade of doctor	Number of patients	%
ST3 or above*	115	65.0
ST2*	31	17.5
Consultant	10	5.6
FY	9	5.1
NCCG	7	4.0
SAS	5	2.8
Subtotal	**177**	
Not applicable	25	
Not answered	46	
Total	**248**	

For the purpose of these data ST3 was equivalent to SpR3 and ST2 equivalent to SpR1-2

The Advisors were asked to determine from the case notes whether the prescription contained adequate information for the nursing staff to deliver the PN safely. In 59 cases the prescription could not be found in the case notes. Of the remaining 205 cases 12 (5.9%) cases were identified as having inadequate detail (Table 3.21).

The constituents of PN can be formulated using a variety of different methods. These may be in the form of bespoke solutions that are tailored to the patient's requirements and these are generally prepared under sterile conditions in the pharmacy. Alternatively, standard formulations are available that can be taken "off the shelf" with or without the addition of other PN additives. Regardless of the methods of formulation employed, uncritical review of the constituents of PN may be detrimental to growth and development. In this study while the single most common method was bespoke, standard formulations of one form or another were used in approximately equal measure (Table 3.22).

Table 3.21 Adequacy of prescription for nurses

Prescription adequate	Number of patients	%
Yes	193	94.1
No	12	5.9
Subtotal	205	
Insufficient data	59	
Total	264	

Table 3.22 Type of PN first administered

Type of PN	Number of patients	%
Multi chamber bag (off the shelf)	36	15.3
Multi chamber bag and additives	34	14.4
Bespoke	86	36.4
Single chamber	37	15.7
Other	21	8.9
Not documented	22	9.3
Subtotal	236	
Insufficient data	28	
Total	264	

Table 3.23 Advisors' opinion on the adequacy of the first PN for the patients' needs

PN adequate	Number of patients	%
Yes	112	62.9
No	66	37.1
Subtotal	178	
Unknown/insufficient data	86	
Total	264	

The Advisors reviewed the case notes to determine whether in their opinion the PN constituents were adequate for the needs of the neonate (Table 3.23). In 66/178 (37.1%) of cases they considered that this was not the case, however in 86 cases there was insufficient information in the case notes to form an opinion. The inadequacy of PN did not appear to be dependant on the type of PN formulation employed (Figure 3.4). The commonly cited reasons for inadequate PN constituents were insufficient amino acid and lipid content or too slow progression of these constituents.

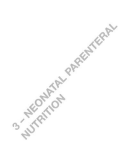

Number of Patients

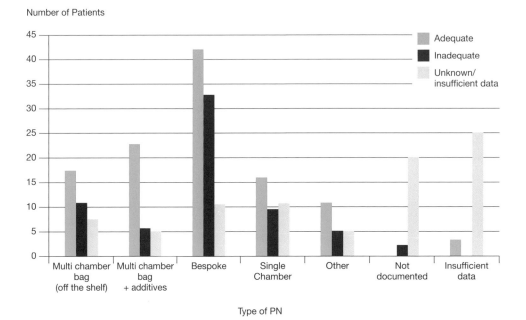

Type of PN

Figure 3.4 Type of PN first administered and the Advisors' opinion on the adequacy of its constituents for the patient's needs

This being the case one has to question why nearly 40% of neonates included in this study did not receive adequate PN for their needs? This is in the face of both guidelines and scientific evidence that in extremely low birth weight neonates' growth outcome is improved if PN is started soon after birth so that the full nutritional value can be achieved early in postnatal life. It is possible that some neonatologists in many neonatal units still hold the traditional view that delayed or more gradual progression of amino acid and lipid content of PN is best practice. Regardless of whether this is true, there should be greater consensus on best PN practice within the neonatal units in the UK.

Administration

It should be possible to commence PN at any time of the day or any day of the week. However this will be dependent on the availability of the healthcare professionals involved in PN particularly the dispensing pharmacist. In this study there was little difference in the number of cases when PN was started based on the days of the week, except for Sunday, which had the lowest frequency (Table 3.24). The majority of PN was commenced out of hours (Table 3.25). The Advisors considered that administration of PN commenced at a reasonable time of day in the majority of cases (Table 3.26).

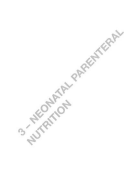
Table 3.24 Day of the week on which PN was commenced

Day PN commenced	Number of patients	%
Monday	45	18.7
Tuesday	33	13.7
Wednesday	33	13.7
Thursday	39	16.2
Friday	38	15.8
Saturday	33	13.7
Sunday	20	8.3
Subtotal	**241**	
Unknown	23	
Total	**264**	

Table 3.25 Time of day on which PN was commenced

Time PN commenced	Number of patients	%
00:00 – 07:59	22	12.7
08:00 – 18:00	45	26.0
18:01 – 23:59	106	61.3
Subtotal	**173**	
Unknown	91	
Total	**264**	

Table 3.26 Advisors' view on whether PN was commenced at a reasonable time of day

Reasonable time	Number of patients	%
Yes	180	96.8
No	6	3.2
Subtotal	**186**	
Unknown/insufficient data	78	
Total	**264**	

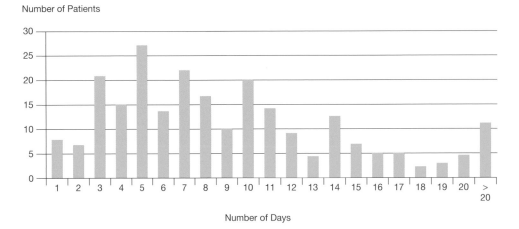

Number of Patients

Number of Days

Figure 3.5 Number of days for which PN was received

Table 3.27 Patient outcome (clinician questionnaire)

Patient outcome	Number of patients	%
Weaned on to oral/enteral feeding	127	51.2
Weaned on to oral/enteral feeding, discharged home	37	14.9
Discharged home	23	9.3
Transferred to different unit	24	9.7
Died during hospital	22	8.9
Weaned, transferred to other unit	10	4.0
Home PN	1	<1
Other	4	1.6
Total	**248**	

During the data collection period the majority of neonates received PN for less than two weeks duration and were successfully weaned on to enteral feeds (Figure 3.5 and Table 3.27).

Clinical and Biochemical Review

Once PN has commenced it is an essential requirement that each neonate has regular and adequate clinical and biochemical review of their nutritional status. This is important to ensure that their needs are met by the PN administered and to avoid complications.

As most of the neonates in this study were cared for on a neonatal unit, one would expect that there would be good evidence from the case notes of frequent clinical reviews. This was indeed found to be the case as shown in Table 3.28. Most of these reviews were undertaken at a senior level (Table 3.29).

Despite this finding, when the Advisors were asked about the adequacy of monitoring of PN they identified 44/226 (19.5%) cases in which they considered monitoring inadequate (Table 3.30). The deficiencies identified were multiple and are shown in Figure 3.6. It seems that some basic monitoring was not undertaken in many neonates in relation to review of PN constitution, or biochemical investigation including glucose and fluid balance.

This raises the question of the adequacy and detail of consideration and knowledge applied to PN during the clinical reviews by senior neonatologists.

Table 3.28 Advisors' views on whether the frequency of reviews was adequate

Adequate frequency of reviews	Number of patients	%
Yes	250	96.9
No	8	3.1
Subtotal	258	
Unknown/insufficient data	6	
Total	264	

Table 3.29 Advisors' views on whether the number of senior reviews was adequate

Senior reviews adequate	Number of patients	%
Yes	129	92.1
No	11	7.9
Subtotal	140	
Unknown/insufficient data	124	
Total	264	

Table 3.30 Advisors' opinion on the adequacy of clinical and biochemical monitoring

Adequate monitoring	Number of patients	%
Yes	182	80.5
No	44	19.5
Subtotal	226	
Unknown/insufficient data	38	
Total	264	

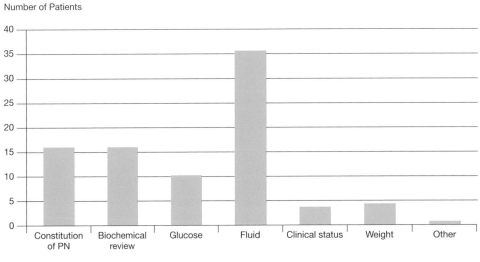

Number of Patients

Deficiencies in Monitoring

Figure 3.6 Deficiencies in clinical and biochemical monitoring (answers may be multiple)

Metabolic Complications

Apart from the complications related to the route of vascular access (see Chapter 4), complications due to the administration of PN can result in metabolic derangement. These include deficiency or excess of individual nutritional constituents of PN e.g. electrolytes, glucose, fatty acids, vitamins and trace elements. Avoiding these complications is essential in providing safe PN care.

The Advisors were asked, from reviewing the case notes, to establish if any metabolic complications had occurred. They found in 63/207 (30.4%) of neonates that this had been the case (Table 3.31). They were further asked to identify the nature of these complications which are shown in Figure 3.7. Not only were there a large number of complications, but it is of considerable concern that of these complications 25 were deemed to be avoidable (Table 3.32), and in 12 neonates complications were not managed appropriately in the view of the Advisors (Table 3.33).

Table 3.31 Evidence of metabolic complications

Metabolic complications	Number of patients	%
Yes	63	30.4
No	144	69.6
Subtotal	**207**	
Insufficient data	57	
Total	**264**	

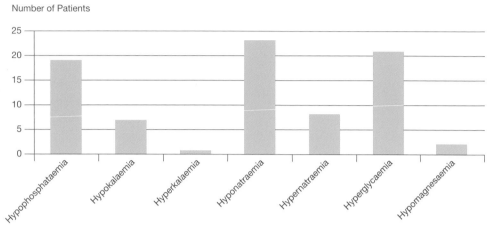

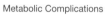

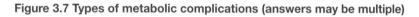

Figure 3.7 Types of metabolic complications (answers may be multiple)

Table 3.32 Advisors' opinion on whether the metabolic complications that developed were avoidable

Metabolic complications avoidable	Number of patients
Yes	25
No	19
Subtotal	**44**
Unknown/insufficient data	19
Total	**63**

Table 3.33 Advisors' opinion on whether the metabolic complications that developed were managed appropriately

Managed appropriately	Number of patients
Yes	33
No	12
Subtotal	**45**
Unknown/insufficient data	18
Total	**63**

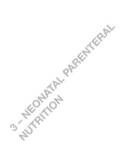

The Advisors frequently commented that there was a large variation in neonatal PN practice in relation to nutritional requirements, prescribing, and constituents of PN bags. Furthermore there was insufficient attention paid to detail with regard to fluid balance, monitoring and review of PN care - all of which led to complications which were not always recognised by the neonatal team and could have resulted in catastrophic outcomes. In 18 neonates where metabolic complications were avoidable, 15 were judged by the Advisors to have had inappropriate PN for their needs (Figure 3.8). Again this reflects the lack of consideration and knowledge applied to PN care.

Examples of inadequate PN included:
• Inadequate sodium content of PN which resulted in hyponatraemia
• Low serum sodium clearly documented but no additional sodium given in PN in situations of both normal and increased sodium losses
• Hypernatraemia due to additional sodium given by a non PN route

• Hyperglycaemia due to too high glucose load both due to excess of glucose in PN and by an alternative administration, not always treated adequately
• Inadequate phosphate content in standard PN bag if appropriate monitoring had occurred low serum phosphate could have been avoided
• Despite low phosphate noted by neonatal team no additional phosphate given in PN

Additional intravenous fluids

Great care needs to be taken in managing fluid balance in sick or premature neonates. Whether the neonate is given sole or supplementary PN, on occasions additional intravenous fluids may be required. The additional intravenous fluid may be accommodated within the PN prescription, however, this is not always possible depending on the clinical state of the infant. Consequently additional intravenous fluids may need to be administered separately to the PN.

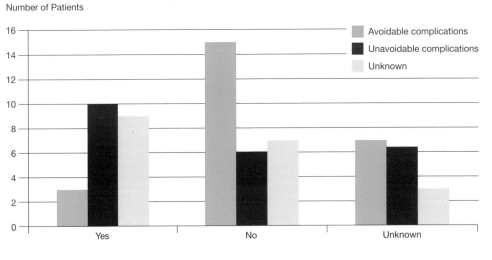

Figure 3.8 Adequacy of PN and whether the metabolic complications that developed were avoidable – Advisors' opinion

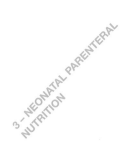

In this sample of neonates additional intravenous fluids were given at some point in 134/238 (56.3%) of cases (Table 3.34). In 11 neonates the type of fluid given was judged by the Advisors to be appropriate (Table 3.35). The volume of additional intravenous fluids given was considered to be inappropriate in nine neonates (Table 3.36).

The Advisors identified situations where neonates should have received a greater PN volume rather than additional intravenous fluids, where additional sodium should have been added to PN, not via separate infusion and where excessive 10% glucose was given in addition to PN leading to hyperglycaemia. Furthermore there were examples of excessive volumes of additional intravenous fluids being given which resulted in a significant positive balance in ventilatory dependant infants.

Table 3.34 Evidence of additional IV fluids given

Fluids given	Number of patients	%
Yes	134	56.3
No	104	43.7
Subtotal	238	
Insufficient data	26	
Total	264	

Table 3.35 Advisors' opinion on the appropriateness of the type of additional fluid

Appropriate fluids	Number of patients	%
Yes	116	91.3
No	11	8.7
Subtotal	127	
Insufficient data	7	
Total	134	

Table 3.36 Advisors' opinion on the appropriateness of the volume of additional fluid

Volume appropriate	Number of patients	%
Yes	91	91.0
No	9	9.0
Subtotal	100	
Insufficient data	34	
Total	134	

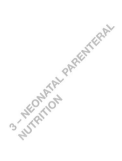

Key Findings

- Good practice in PN care was identified in only 24% (62/264) of the neonates in this study.
- There were delays in recognising the need for PN in 28% (71/252) of neonates and a delay in starting PN once the decision to commence PN had been made in 17% (36/210) of the neonates.
- The requirements for PN were only documented in 28% (70/250) of patients.
- In 37% (66/178) of neonates the first PN provided was considered inadequate for the patient's needs.
- While the majority of neonates had an appropriate level of senior review, in 19% (44/226) of cases the monitoring of PN was deemed inadequate. Basic monitoring was not undertaken in many neonates in relation to review of PN constitution, biochemical investigation including glucose and fluid balance.
- In 63 neonates metabolic complications related to PN were identified which were considered avoidable in 25 and managed inappropriately in 12.
- There are guidelines and scientific evidence that in extremely low birth weight neonates' growth outcome is improved if PN is started soon after birth so that the full nutritional value can be achieved early in postnatal life. These are not followed by some neonatal units where there are delays in the introduction and rate of progression of the amino acid and lipid content of PN.
- There was a large variation in neonatal PN practice in relation to nutritional requirements, prescribing, and constituents of PN bags. Furthermore there was not enough attention to detail paid to fluid balance, monitoring and review of PN care. All of which led to complications which were not always recognised by the neonatal team and could have resulted in catastrophic outcomes.

Recommendations

- Careful and early consideration should be given to the need for PN in neonates and once the decision to commence PN is made it should be started without undue delay. (Consultants)
- The first PN given must be appropriate to the neonate's requirements. (Consultants)
- Close monitoring of the patient must be achieved so that metabolic complications can be avoided. (Consultants)
- Neonatal Units should have an agreed policy for nutritional requirements and use a proforma that includes this information which is tailored for each infant and placed in the case notes. (Clinical Directors)
- Hospitals in which neonates are cared for should develop a team approach to ensure safe and effective nutritional support, recognising that this should be a multidisciplinary exercise with sharing of expertise. Depending on the type of institution and availability of personnel, the composition of these teams may vary but could include neonatologists, paediatricians, paediatric surgeons, pharmacists, dietitions and experts in nutrition. This team could also provide support to other clinical areas caring for children and have a role in education and training for those involved in PN care. (Medical Directors)
- There is an urgent need for Neonatal Units across the UK to have a consensus on best PN practice based on current scientific evidence. (Consultant Neonatologists)
- Neonatal units should undertaken regular audit of PN practice which should include the complications of PN. (Clinical Directors)
- The National Institute for Health and Clinical Excellence should develop guidelines on nutritional support for neonates and children in a similar manner to their recommendations for adults. (NICE)

Parenteral nutrition (PN) is administered via an intravenous feeding catheter, usually a central venous catheter (CVC). Administration via a central route is preferable as PN has the potential to cause thrombosis/phlebitis if given peripherally. CVCs come in several different types which vary both according to their site of insertion and the type of device used; the choice being dependant upon the indication for the PN, as different expected lengths of treatment require different devices. It is important that all CVCs are inserted by a suitably trained clinician under appropriate sterile conditions. Once inserted the position of the CVC should be checked with a plain radiograph or ultrasound (in neonates). Following insertion it is important that the CVC is cared for appropriately: the key elements being that it should be used only for PN ('dedicated catheter'); only accessed by individuals trained in the use and care of CVCs; and accessed as little as possible. In this way the risk of infection is reduced. Infection of CVCs is a cause of major morbidity and potentially fatal. In adults CVC

infections are also notoriously difficult to clear. There are other inherent risks associated with CVCs, many of which are avoidable if the catheter is inserted under the right conditions and appropriately looked after.

Adults

The type of cannulation device used to administer PN as reported by the clinicians is shown in Table 4.1; the commonest being a centrally inserted venous catheter. This represented 762/1042 (73%) of the cases within the study. However it should be noted that the clinicians did not return these data in 290 cases. Of the CVCs inserted 751 were multilumen (cuffed/uncuffed) and 283 single lumen (uncuffed/cuffed) (Table 4.2). The clinicians reported that only 42% were inserted solely for PN. It should be noted that 127 patients received their first PN via a peripheral catheter which is not ideal and may precipitate phlebitis.

Table 4.1 Initial mode of PN delivery

PN delivery	Number of patients	%
Centrally inserted venous catheter	449	43.1
Centrally inserted venous catheter – non-tunelled	237	22.7
Centrally inserted venous catheter – tunnelled	76	7.3
Peripherally inserted central venous catheter	153	14.7
Peripheral venous catheter	127	12.2
Subtotal	1042	
Unknown/not answered	290	
Total	1332	

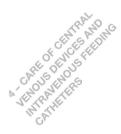

Table 4.2 Initial type of PN catheter

Type of catheter	Number of patients	%
Multilumen	673	65.1
Multilumen uncuffed	60	5.8
Multilumen cuffed	18	1.7
Single lumen	241	23.3
Single lumen cuffed	24	2.3
Single lumen uncuffed	18	1.7
Subtotal	1034	
Unknown/not answered	298	
Total	1332	

Table 4.3 Catheter insertion site documented in the case notes

Insertion site documented	Number of patients	%
Yes	554	67.4
No	268	32.6
Subtotal	822	
Insufficient data	55	
Total	877	

Table 4.4 Catheter insertion site appropriate – Advisors' opinion

Insertion site appropriate	Number of patients	%
Yes	508	95.1
No	26	4.9
Subtotal	534	
Insufficient data	20	
Total	554	

The Advisors found that 268/822 (32.6%) of adult patients did not have any documentation of the site of the feeding catheter inserted (Table 4.3). As a highly invasive procedure, fraught with potential complications it is disappointing that documentation was so poor. However where documentation was found (Table 4.4), the recorded site of catheter insertion was appropriate in the view of the advisors in the vast majority of patients (95.1%).

Approximately three quarters of adult patients (612/837) were found by the Advisors to have had the type of feeding catheter inserted recorded (as opposed to the

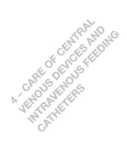

documentation of insertion); and in 90% (537/597) this was deemed an appropriate device for the anticipated type and duration of PN as judged by the Advisors (Tables 4.5 and 4.6). However this still leaves 60 patients who were administered PN through a feeding catheter judged to be inappropriate by the Advisors with all the complications that this can engender.

When a CVC is employed it is of clinical importance that the position of its tip is documented as this acts as a record of insertion of the tip to an appropriate anatomical position; ideally this should be in the lower third of the Superior Vena Cava or at the junction of the Superior Vena Cava and right atrium. The upper right atrium is also acceptable. Appropriate tip position has been shown to reduce CVC complications[18]. The position was not recorded in over half the adult patients (377/692; Table 4.7). The Advisors believe that a failure to record this information may have heightened the risk of mechanical/thrombotic complications owing to unrecognised CVC misplacement.

Table 4.5 Type of catheter documented in the case notes

Type of catheter documented	Number of patients	%
Yes	612	73.1
No	225	26.9
Subtotal	**837**	
Insufficient data	40	
Total	**877**	

Table 4.6 Type of catheter appropriate – Advisors' opinion

Type of catheter appropriate	Number of patients	%
Yes	537	89.9
No	60	10.1
Subtotal	**597**	
Insufficient data	15	
Total	**612**	

Table 4.7 Position of tip documented in the case notes

Position of tip documented	Number of patients	%
Yes	315	45.5
No	377	54.5
Subtotal	**692**	
Not applicable	62	
Insufficient data	123	
Total	**877**	

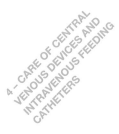
As previously mentioned it is of importance that the CVC is a dedicated catheter and used for PN only with minimal access to it. This reduces the risk of catheter infection which is a cause of serious morbidity and mortality. The Advisors found that in 50/648 (7.7%) of patients there was evidence of inappropriate CVC care (Table 4.8). In over a third of patients (224/605) the CVC was being used for purposes other than PN (Table 4.9). They found in this group that CVCs were being accessed for the administration of supplemental IV fluids, blood products and drug administration. This is unacceptable as the risk of infection and complications will increase if the CVC is not single purpose.

There was a high incidence of CVC complications in this study group. The Advisors were of the opinion that 26% (193/734) of CVCs were associated with complications (Table 4.10) - the commonest of these being suspected or confirmed catheter infections (Figure 4.1). It is perhaps a matter of debate whether a suspected catheter infection can be classified as a true complication; but if all other sources of sepsis have been excluded it is highly indicative of catheter related sepsis.

Table 4.8 Evidence of inappropriate CVC care

Inappropriate CVC care	Number of patients	%
Yes	50	7.7
No	598	92.3
Subtotal	648	
Insufficient data	229	
Total	877	

Table 4.9 Evidence of additional CVC usage

CVC use other than PN	Number of patients	%
Yes	224	37.0
No	381	63.0
Subtotal	605	
Insufficient data	272	
Total	877	

Table 4.10 Evidence of CVC complications

CVC complications	Number of patients	%
Yes	193	26.3
No	541	73.7
Subtotal	734	
Insufficient data	143	
Total	877	

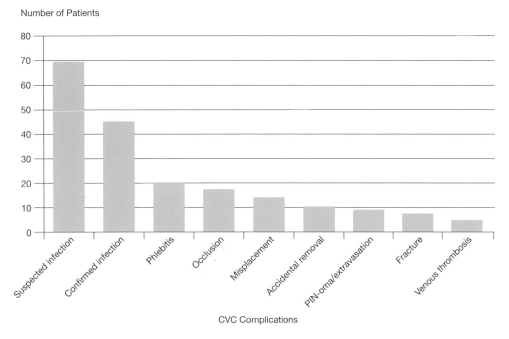

Number of Patients

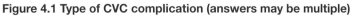

CVC Complications

Figure 4.1 Type of CVC complication (answers may be multiple)

In an ideal world complications would never occur; however when they do they should have been unforeseeable and/or unavoidable. The Advisors judged that over half (55/102) of all CVC-related complications were avoidable (Table 4.11). This is a striking figure as it suggests a lack of awareness that these complications could occur, a lack of surveillance of the possible complications or worse, complacency. As CVC related complications are by definition iatrogenic, it is unconscionable for avoidable complications to be allowed to happen. The unacceptability of this finding is further compounded by the Advisors opining that 12% (20/165) of all complications were managed inappropriately (Table 4.12). Thus some complications have been found to be both avoidable and even when not avoidable some were managed badly.

Table 4.11 Advisors' opinion on whether the CVC complications were avoidable

Complications avoidable	Number of patients	%
Yes	55	53.9
No	47	46.1
Subtotal	102	
Unknown	91	
Total	193	

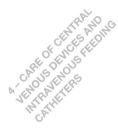

Table 4.12 Advisors' opinion on whether the CVC complications were managed appropriately

Complications managed appropriately	Number of patients	%
Yes	145	87.9
No	20	12.1
Subtotal	**165**	
Unknown	28	
Total	**193**	

Table 4.13 Evidence of CVC and/or metabolic complications

CVC complication(s)	Metabolic complications				Total
	Yes	No	Subtotal	Insufficient data	
Yes	65	73	**138**	55	**193**
No	148	269	**417**	124	**541**
Subtotal	**213**	**342**	**555**	**179**	**734**
Insufficient data	36	43	**79**	64	**143**
Total	**249**	**385**	**634**	**243**	**877**

Table 4.14 Initial mode of PN delivery – clinician questionnaire

PN delivery	Number of patients	%
Peripheral venous catheter	41	17.4
Peripherally inserted central venous catheter	109	46.2
Umbilical vein	69	29.2
Centrally inserted venous catheter	17	7.2
Subtotal	**236**	
Not answered	12	
Total	**248**	

Table 4.13 shows the occurrence of CVC-related and metabolic complications. As can be seen 65/555 (11.7%) of patients developed both a metabolic and CVC-related complication. Furthermore, over half of the adult patients (286/555) in the study developed a catheter and/or metabolic complication and in 91 there was insufficient data to assess. This is both unfortunate and may suggest a generally poor standard of both catheter and PN care.

Neonates

Within the neonatal group, the clinicians completing the clinician questionnaire were asked the initial mode of PN delivery. One can see that the most commonly employed technique was a peripherally inserted central venous catheter (Table 4.14). Documentation of the site of line insertion and the type of catheter inserted could only be

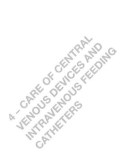

determined from the case notes in 183/246 (74.4%) and 167/250 (66.8%) of neonates respectively (Tables 4.15 and 4.17). Where there was documentation, in the majority of cases the site of insertion and type of catheter was deemed appropriate by the Advisors (Tables 4.16 and 4.18).

Table 4.15 Catheter insertion site documented in the case notes

Site of insertion documented	Number of patients	%
Yes	183	74.4
No	63	25.6
Subtotal	246	
Insufficient data	18	
Total	264	

Table 4.16 Catheter insertion site appropriate – Advisors' opinion

Insertion site appropriate	Number of patients	%
Yes	174	96.1
No	7	3.9
Subtotal	181	
Insufficient data	2	
Total	183	

Table 4.17 Type of catheter documented in the case notes

Type of catheter documented	Number of patients	%
Yes	167	66.8
No	83	33.2
Subtotal	250	
Insufficient data	14	
Total	264	

Table 4.18 Type of Catheter appropriate – Advisors' opinion

Type of catheter appropriate	Number of patients	%
Yes	155	93.9
No	10	6.1
Subtotal	165	
Insufficient data	2	
Total	167	

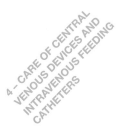

As can be seen the position of the tip of the catheter was documented in 62.2% of cases (Table 4.19) and the position appropriate in 86.4% of these (Table 4.20).

The evidence for inappropriate catheter care and use of the catheter for purposes other than PN largely reflects the adult data (Tables 4.21 and 4.22). Within the neonatal group the catheter was used for purposes other than PN in over a third (68/191) of cases, and 10 cases (5%) had evidence of inappropriate care. The Advisors believe that this may heighten the risk of infection in neonates although they accept that venous access may be at a premium and thus it may be acceptable to use the feeding catheter for other purposes.

Table 4.19 Position of tip documented in the case notes

Position of tip documented	Number of patients	%
Yes	130	62.2
No	79	37.8
Subtotal	**209**	
Insufficient data	55	
Total	**264**	

Table 4.20 Position of tip appropriate – Advisors' opinion

Position of tip appropriate	Number of patients	%
Yes	95	86.4
No	15	13.6
Subtotal	**110**	
Insufficient data	20	
Total	**130**	

Table 4.21 Evidence of inappropriate CVC care

Inappropriate CVC care	Number of patients	%
Yes	10	5.1
No	188	94.9
Subtotal	**198**	
Insufficient data	66	
Total	**264**	

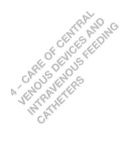

Table 4.22 Evidence of additional CVC usage

CVC use other than PN	Number of patients	%
Yes	68	35.6
No	123	64.4
Subtotal	191	
Insufficient data	73	
Total	264	

Approximately a quarter (56/226) of neonates in this study had complications related directly to their catheter (Table 4.23) and as with the adults this seemed predominantly to relate to suspected or confirmed catheter infections (Figure 4.2). However it should be noted that nine patients had catheter misplacement and seven had extravasation of PN. Furthermore the Advisors found that the complications were avoidable for 6/32 cases (Table 4.24).

Table 4.23 Evidence of CVC complications

CVC complications	Number of patients	%
Yes	56	24.8
No	170	75.2
Subtotal	226	
Insufficient data	38	
Total	264	

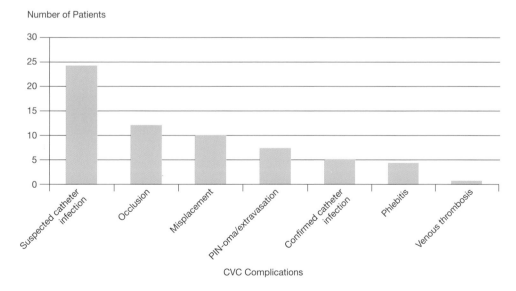

Figure 4.2 Type of CVC complication (answers may be multiple)

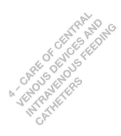
Table 4.24 Advisors' opinion on whether the CVC complications were avoidable

Complications avoidable	Number of patients
Yes	6
No	26
Subtotal	**32**
Unknown	24
Total	**56**

Summary

The data shown provide clear evidence of poor care especially with respect to documentation of catheter insertion and the prevalence of complications (many of which were avoidable). The degree to which catheter care has been shown to be unsatisfactory is marked and suggests that all hospitals should have clear policies with respect to the insertion of CVCs/catheters. This should include clear documentation as to the type and site of catheter insertion including tip position. There should be education around the possible complications of CVCs leading to a greater understanding and surveillance for these complications. These policies should be patient-specific (adults/neonates) and not all encompassing global documents. The prevalence, avoidability and management of catheter complications in each patient group (adults/neonates) should be made, illustrated and emphasised. This approach would reduce the risk of complications both in adult and neonatal practice.

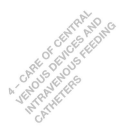

Key Findings

- Lack of adequate documentation of catheter site insertion in a third (268/822) of adults and in 26% (63/246) of neonates.
- Position of tip of catheter not documented in 55% (377/692) of adults and 38% (79/209) of neonates.
- Catheter complications occurred in 26% (193/734) of adults and 25% (56/226) of neonates.
- Complications were avoidable in 54% (55/102) of adults and 6/32 of neonates.
- 12% (20/165) of adult complications not managed appropriately in the view of the Advisors.
- 58% (377/646) of adults in this study had a catheter and/or metabolic complication.

Recommendations

- CVC insertion is an invasive procedure with well recognised risks. Insertion should be clearly documented in the case notes including:
  - The designation of the operator
  - The type of CVC
  - A description of the insertion technique
  - The use of imaging
  - Confirmation of the position of the catheter tip
  (Consultants)
- All hospitals must have policies on the management CVCs which should include:
  - Insertion of CVC
  - Care of indwelling CVC
  - Detection and management of complications
  - Monitoring and audit, including adherence to the policies
  (Medical Directors)
- There must be improved education around CVC insertion and management; as well as the recognition and management of CVC complications.
  (Clinical Directors)

5 – Organisational Data

An Organisational Questionnaire was sent to each hospital believed to provide PN. This section of the report covers the facilities, policies, and procedures adopted when providing PN.

Adult Organisational Data

Once the decision to administer PN has been made, it is of vital importance that the composition is accurately determined so the nutritional needs of the patient are met and the risk of metabolic complications minimised.

Table 5.1 shows the members of staff that were responsible for determining the composition of PN on adult wards during the study period.

There was little difference between wards in the type of staff responsible for determining PN composition and whether or not they would usually belong to a nutrition team (Figures 5.1 and 5.2).

Table 5.1 Designation of the person responsible for deciding on the PN composition on adult wards

Designation	Type of adult ward		
	Medical	**Surgical**	**ICU**
Medical staff/Dietitian/Pharmacist/Nutrition Nurse Specialist	20	21	19
Medical staff/Dietitian/Pharmacist	40	38	43
Medical staff/Dietitian	21	20	18
Medical staff/Dietitian/Nutrition Nurse Specialist	2	2	1
Medical staff/Pharmacist/Nutrition Nurse Specialist	2	2	1
Medical staff/Pharmacist	6	6	9
Medical staff	13	11	20
Dietitian/Pharmacist/Nutrition Nurse Specialist	12	12	10
Dietitian/Pharmacist	31	33	23
Dietitian/Nutrition Nurse Specialist	3	3	2
Dietitian	35	33	23
Pharmacist/Nutrition Nurse Specialist	1	1	1
Pharmacist	8	8	6
Total	**194**	**190**	**176**

Number of Hospitals

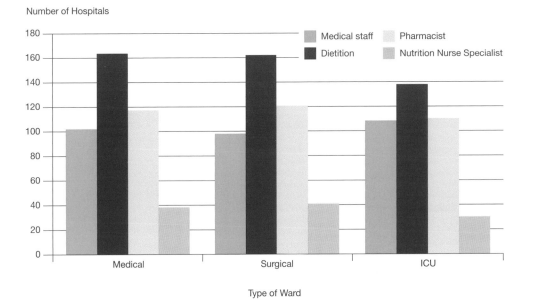

Type of Ward

Figure 5.1 Who decides on PN composition by type on adult wards

Number of Hospitals

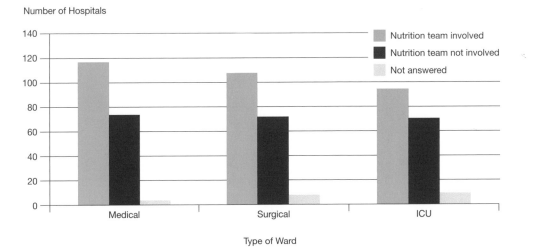

Type of Ward

Figure 5.2 Nutritional team involvement in determining PN composition on adult wards

Table 5.2 Designation of the person responsible for prescribing PN on adult wards

Designation	Type of adult ward		
	Medical	Surgical	ICU
Medical staff	141	137	132
Medical staff/Pharmacist	22	23	20
Medical staff/Pharmacist/Nutrition Nurse Specialist	4	4	2
Medical staff/Pharmacist/Nutrition Nurse Specialist/Dietitian	2	3	3
Medical staff/Nutrition Nurse Specialist/Dietitian	0	1	1
Medical staff/Nutrition Nurse Specialist	5	3	3
Medical staff/Dietitian	6	6	3
Medical staff/Pharmacist/Dietitian	4	4	4
Pharmacist	7	6	6
Pharmacist/Nutrition Nurse Specialist	2	1	1
Pharmacist/Nutrition Nurse Specialist/Dietitian	0	1	1
Nutrition Nurse Specialist/Dietitian	1	1	0
Total	**194**	**190**	**176**

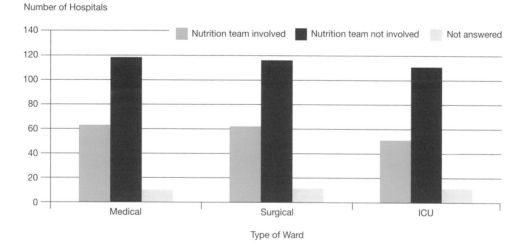

Figure 5.3 Nutritional team involvement in prescribing PN on adult wards

The job of prescribing PN was predominantly undertaken by medical staff (Table 5.2) and involved a member of the nutrition team in about a third of hospitals (Figure 5.3). Whilst this suggests that the person signing the PN prescription will often not have been involved in determining its composition, the significance of this is unknown as it may reflect the legal necessity that a doctor's signature is required.

Number of Hospitals

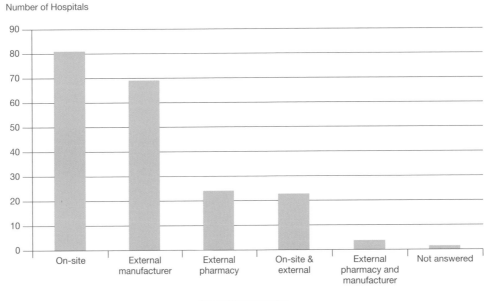

Site of PN Preparation

Figure 5.4 Adult PN preparation

Approximately half of the hospitals in the study had PN prepared on-site (Figure 5.4) and all bar 18 (9%) were able to obtain tailored bags/bags with additives from their pharmacy/manufacturer (Table 5.3). The availability of bespoke bags tended to be limited to weekdays (162/184 hospitals; Table 5.4) which is in line with the opening times of pharmacies and external manufacturers.

Table 5.3 Bespoke bags produced by pharmacy/manufacturer

Bespoke bags	Number of hospitals	%
Yes	184	91.1
No	18	8.9
Total	**202**	

Table 5.4 Availability of bespoke bags

Bespoke bags	Number of hospitals	%
7 days/week	15	8.2
5 days/week	162	88.0
Other	7	3.8
Total	**184**	

Table 5.5 Maintenance of PN stock

PN stock on ward	Number of hospitals	%
Yes	68	34.5
No	129	65.5
Subtotal	**197**	
Not answered	5	
Total	**202**	

Whilst PN is not an emergency intervention for adults, it is desirable to have a short turn around time for PN so it can be commenced or continued the same day it is known to be needed. The PN turn around time for the large majority of hospitals in this study (177/199; 89%) was the same day if it was ordered within normal working hours (Figure 5.5).

The current study found that approximately a third of hospitals (68/197) maintained stocks of PN on particular wards, most notably on Level 3 (Tables 5.5 and 5.6). Whilst this was of concern to some of the Experts and Advisors, the type of PN maintained in ward stocks was not explored, so it is unknown whether this could contribute to patients receiving inappropriate PN. However, of immediate concern was the finding that 27 of the hospitals that maintained stocks of PN on specific wards, did not maintain a central record of the patients receiving this PN (Table 5.7).

Number of Hospitals

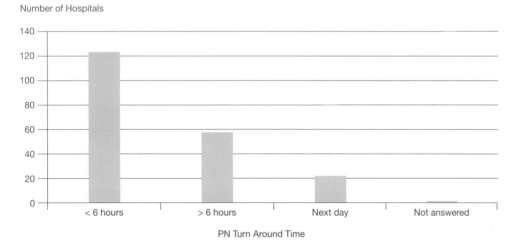
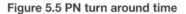

PN Turn Around Time

Figure 5.5 PN turn around time

Table 5.6 Type of wards that maintain PN stocks

Type of ward	Number of hospitals
Level 3	52
Surgical ward/Level 3	8
Medical ward/Surgical ward/Level 3	3
Surgical ward	3
Subtotal	**66**
Not answered	2
Total	**68**

Table 5.7 Central record of PN stocks

Central record kept	Number of hospitals
Yes	39
No	27
Subtotal	**66**
Not answered	2
Total	**68**

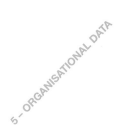

Nutrition Teams

To achieve safe administration of PN to patients where this method of nutrition is indicated, it would seem logical to adopt a co-ordinated team approach. It was therefore disappointing to find that 40% (80/201) of hospitals that administer PN to adult patients did not have a nutrition team (Table 5.8).

Table 5.8 Presence of a nutrition team for adult patients

Nutrition team	Number of hospitals	%
Yes	121	60.2
No	80	39.8
Subtotal	201	
Not answered	1	
Total	202	

When the overall PN-related care was correlated with whether nutrition teams were involved in the initial decision to give PN there was a difference seen in the good practice and less than satisfactory categories but very little difference in the middle ground represented by the other categories (Table 5.9). This may be because nutrition teams were only involved at the outset rather than all the way through the process, although this seems unlikely. Further data analysis could not identify a clear benefit of nutrition teams in terms of good overall care but this probably reflects the fact that the Advisors were grading care on a large number of parameters not just whether nutrition teams made a difference. Mindful of this, NCEPOD would support a multidisciplinary team approach to PN to ensure that there is an overarching monitoring process in the initiation and administration of PN.

The specialties of the doctors belonging to the nutrition teams are shown in Table 5.10. Despite the fact that surgical patients were the largest group receiving PN in this study (see Chapter 2), there was a very low involvement of surgeons in nutrition teams. This may reflect a lack of professional interest in nutrition amongst surgeons coupled with a readiness to delegate these duties to dietitians, nurses and gastroenterologists.

Table 5.9 Nutrition team involvement in the decision to give PN and overall assessment of PN care (data from Advisor assessment form and clinician questionnaire)

	Nutrition team involved in the decision to give PN			
	Yes		No	
Overall Assessment	Number of patients	%	Number of patients	%
Good practice	101	27.4	49	15.2
Room for improvement - clinical	124	33.6	118	36.6
Room for improvement - organisational	37	10.0	36	11.2
Room for improvement - clinical and organisational	81	22.0	82	25.5
Less than satisfactory	26	7.0	37	11.5
Total	369		322	

Table 5.10 Specialties of doctors belonging to nutrition teams (answers may be multiple)

Specialty	Number of hospitals
Gastroenterology	95
General or Chemical pathology	17
Colorectal surgery	7
General surgery	7
Anaesthetics	4
Critical/intensive care med	4
Other surgery	4
Other medicine	3
No doctor in team	11

Table 5.11 shows the other members of the nutrition teams; 71/121 (59%) had a dietitian, pharmacist and nutrition nurse specialist.

Table 5.11 Nutrition team members

Team members	Number of hospitals
Dietitian/Pharmacist/Nutrition Nurse Specialist/Biochemist	10
Dietitian/Pharmacist/Nutrition Nurse Specialist	61
Dietitian/Pharmacist/Biochemist	2
Dietitian/Pharmacist	31
Dietitian/Nutrition Nurse Specialist	7
Dietitian	7
Pharmacist/Nutrition Nurse Specialist	2
Pharmacist	1
Total	**121**

The 11 teams that did not have a doctor, consisted of a dietitian and pharmacist (7/11 hospitals).

The data were interrogated to identify how often the nutrition team held a multidisciplinary team meeting (MDT). As can be seen in Table 5.12, half (55/110) of the nutrition teams met on a weekly basis. It was also reported that 13 teams rarely or never had an MDT meeting and 11 adopted an as needed approach.

Table 5.12 Frequency of nutrition MDT meeting

Frequency	Number of hospitals
Weekly	55
Fortnightly	1
Monthly	12
Every 2 months	10
Every 3 months	6
2-3 times per year	2
As required	11
Rarely	6
Never	7
Subtotal	**110**
Not answered	11
Total	**121**

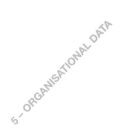
Just under half (55/119) of the teams undertook daily ward rounds, 16/119 on alternate days, whilst the majority of the remainder (30/119) had weekly nutrition team rounds (Table 5.13). NCEPOD believes that MDT meetings and full nutrition team ward rounds should, as a minimum, occur weekly.

Table 5.13 Frequency of nutrition team ward rounds

Frequency	Number of hospitals
Daily (7 days/week)	1
Daily (5 days/week)	54
2-3 days per week	16
Weekly	30
As required	8
Rarely	4
Never	6
Subtotal	119
Not answered	2
Total	121

NCEPOD explored the function of the nutrition teams. As can be seen in Table 5.14, 50/117 (43%) nutrition teams reviewed only PN referrals whilst the remainder 63/108 (58%) saw both PN and enteral nutrition referrals. It is interesting that such a high proportion only saw PN referrals. It is arguable that a truly multi-professional and multipurpose nutrition team should have the capability to see both.

Table 5.14 Function of the nutrition team

Function	Number of hospitals	%
Review only PN referrals	50	42.7
Review enteral & PN referrals	67	57.3
Subtotal	117	
Not answered	4	
Total	121	

Approximately half (62/118) of the nutrition teams in this study had complete autonomy with respect to ordering and administering PN (i.e. could say no to PN; Table 5.15). Given that we have seen from earlier data that it is not unusual for PN to be given inappropriately, NCEPOD believes that more nutrition teams should have more autonomy.

Table 5.15 Involvement of nutrition teams in ordering and administering PN

Ordering and administering PN	Number of hospitals	%
Complete autonomy	62	52.5
Advisory role	56	47.5
Subtotal	118	
Not answered	3	
Total	121	

Neonatal Organisational Data

Tables 5.16 and 5.17 show the members of staff that were responsible for determining the composition of PN on Neonatal Units during the study period. This task was largely undertaken by medical staff (107/115), often in conjunction with pharmacists (60/115). Dietitian and specialist nurse involvement was very limited (14/115 and 1/115 hospitals respectively). When one considers this and the finding that the Advisors were of the opinion that a large number of neonates received PN that was inadequate for their needs (see Chapter 3 Table 3.23 and Figure 3.4), urgent consensus on best practice, particularly composition, for neonatal PN is needed.

Table 5.16 Designation of the person responsible for determining PN composition on Neonatal Units

Designation	Number of hospitals	%
Medical staff/Pharmacist	52	45.2
Medical staff	40	34.8
Medical staff/Dietitian/Pharmacist	8	7.0
Pharmacist	8	7.0
Medical staff/Dietitian	6	5.2
Medical staff/Nutrition Nurse Specialist	1	<1
Subtotal	115	
Not answered	7	
Total	122	

Table 5.17 Designation of the person responsible for determining PN composition on Neonatal Units

Designation	Number of hospitals	%
Medical staff	107	93.0
Pharmacist	68	59.1
Dietitian	14	12.2
Nutrition Nurse Specialist	1	< 1
Not answered	7	

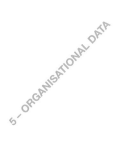

Table 5.18 Designation of the person responsible for prescribing PN on Neonatal Units

Designation	Number of hospitals	%
Medical staff	92	78.6
Medical staff/Pharmacist	20	17.1
Medical staff/Nutrition Nurse Specialist	2	1.7
Pharmacist	2	1.7
Nutrition Nurse Specialist	1	<1
Subtotal	117	
Not answered	5	
Total	122	

Approximately 50% (61/121) of hospitals produced their neonatal PN onsite, whilst 40% (48/121) used an external pharmacy or manufacturer (Figure 5.6). The remaining 10% (12/121) both produced PN onsite and sourced it externally.

Seven hospitals reported that their pharmacy/manufacturer could not supply tailored bags (Table 5.19).

If ordered during normal working hours the turn around time for neonatal PN was < 6 hours for almost two thirds (77/121) of hospitals (Table 5.20). However, it was reported that eight hospitals could not be supplied with PN the same day it was ordered, which is far from ideal for this group of patients. Seven of these hospitals sourced PN from an external manufacturer.

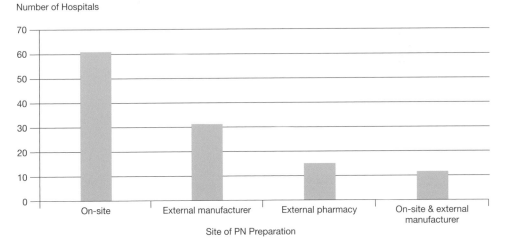

Figure 5.6 Site of neonatal PN preparation

Table 5.19 Production of bespoke bags by pharmacy/manufacturer

Bespoke bags	Number of hospitals	%
Yes	112	94.1
No	7	5.9
Subtotal	119	
Not answered	3	
Total	122	

Table 5.20 PN turn around time

Time	Number of hospitals	%
< 6 hours	77	63.6
> 6 hours but same day	36	29.8
Next day	8	6.6
Subtotal	121	
Not answered	1	
Total	122	

Approximately half of the hospitals kept a stock of PN on Neonatal units (Table 5.21), but 24/58 of these did not maintain a central record of the patients receiving this PN (Table 5.22). As stated in the previous chapter, the Experts and Advisors reviewing the findings were of the opinion that a central record of all patients receiving PN, must be maintained.

Table 5.21 Maintenance of PN stock

PN stock on ward	Number of hospitals	%
Yes	58	48.7
No	61	51.3
Subtotal	119	
Not answered	3	
Total	122	

Table 5.22 Central record of PN stock

Central record kept	Number of hospitals
Yes	34
No	24
Total	58

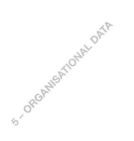
Neonatal Nutrition Teams

Only 15/122 (12%) of hospitals reported that they had a nutrition team that was involved in providing PN support for neonates. The composition of the teams is shown in Table 5.23. The doctors involved in the nutrition teams were mainly neonatologists (8/15) and gastroenterologists (5/15).

Table 5.23 Composition of nutrition teams

Team staff	Number of Hospitals
Doctor/Dietitian	1
Doctor/Dietitian/Pharmacist	8
Doctor/Dietitian/Pharmacist/ Nutrition Nurse Specialist	3
Doctor/Pharmacist	2
Not answered	1
Total	**15**

The majority of neonates included in this study were cared for on a Neonatal unit and it is clear from this study that most units make decisions regarding nutrition in an autonomous manner. This is perhaps not surprising because much of the nutritional expertise will be concentrated within the Neonatal unit amongst consultant neonatologists and senior nursing staff. However not all neonates are cared for within this environment, for example some surgical neonates will be cared for on paediatric general wards where this level of expertise may not be available. While it may not be possible to care for all neonates and infants in one clinical area there is much to be said for at least concentrating the expertise for the management of PN in neonates to those who have the greatest experience in PN care. Thus it would be valuable in hospitals that care for neonates that a multidisciplinary team approach is used to provide PN. Depending on the type of institution the composition of these teams may vary and could include neonatologists, paediatricians, paediatric surgeons, pharmacists, dietitians and experts in nutrition, depending on availability and interest. This would enable good levels of communication and team working with all those involved in administration of PN to ensure safe and effective nutritional support. These teams could be based in Neonatal units but provide additional support to the general paediatric wards. They should also have a responsibility to provide appropriate education and training for those involved in PN care[14].

Parenteral Nutrition Practice

Data from the Advisor peer review meetings showed that a large number of patients, particularly in the adult group, were given PN when it was not indicated (232/808 patients; see Chapter 2). It would therefore seem very appropriate to have hospital guidelines for initiating PN. As can be seen in Figure 5.7, it was reported that 39/201 hospitals did not have guidelines for initiating PN. This was similar when NCEPOD asked about policies for changing/handling PN bags (38/200) (Figure 5.7).

The large majority of hospitals had a policy for the insertion and clinical care of central venous catheters (192/200), with approximately half having a dedicated insertion service (94/201; Figure 5.8).

The rate of CVC complications, and in particular suspected and confirmed catheter infections, was relatively high in this study (see Chapter 4). Therefore it would seem particularly important to have a hospital policy for the management of CVC infection. As can be seen in Figure 5.8, 33/197 (16.8%) hospitals reported that they did not have such a policy.

ESPEN guidelines indicate that co-administration of antibiotics following insertion does not reduce infective complications[18]. Thus it is surprising to see that 14 hospitals were using this intervention (Table 5.24).

Number of Hospitals

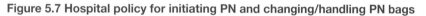

Figure 5.7 Hospital policy for initiating PN and changing/handling PN bags

Number of Hospitals

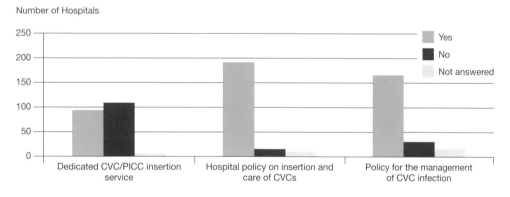

Figure 5.8 Hospital CVC/PICC services and policies

Table 5.24 Use of antibiotic prophylaxis during insertion

Antibiotic prophylaxis used	Number of hospitals	%
Yes	14	7.2
No	180	92.8
Subtotal	**194**	
Not answered	11	
Total	**205**	

Key Findings

- 27 hospitals that supplied adult PN as stock to wards and 24 hospitals that supplied neonatal PN as stock to neonatal units did not have a central record of the patient to whom it was administered.
- 62% of hospitals could provide adult PN and 63% of neonatal PN within 6 hours of request.
- 50 adult nutrition teams saw only PN referrals.
- 81% of hospitals had guidelines on initiating PN.
- 81% of hospitals had guidelines on changing and handling PN bags.
- 53% of hospitals did not have a dedicated CVC/PICC catheter insertion service.
- Despite a high proportion of the patients in the study being surgical there was a very low involvement of surgeons in nutrition teams.

Recommendations

- Nutrition teams have an important role in ensuring quality control around the initiation, supply and monitoring of PN. Whilst the data from this study did not show a clear correlation between overall care and the involvement of a nutrition team it was not designed to do so and no adverse inference should be made from this. All hospitals involved with PN should have a multidisciplinary nutrition team involved in both enteral and parenteral nutrition. (Medical Directors)
- All hospitals should keep a central record of where and to whom PN has been supplied. (Medical Directors and Heads of Pharmacy)
- All hospitals should have policies on initiating PN to avoid inappropriate use and safe prescribing. (Medical Directors)
- All hospitals should have a dedicated CVC/PICC service to ensure high-level expertise is practised within this interventional area. (Medical Directors)
- Surgical teams are high volume users of PN. As such they need to engage more in clinical nutrition issues and increase their profile within nutrition teams. (Medical Directors and Clinical Directors)

Parenteral Nutrition in Children

Only 70 sets of paediatric case notes were received for the Advisor peer review meetings. As a consequence only limited analysis has been undertaken of the information collected.

Parenteral nutrition (PN) in children outside the neonatal period is indicated due to complete or partial intestinal failure from conditions that are a continuation of neonatal causes (either congenital or acquired) or conditions that present during childhood. Parenteral nutrition may be required for short term nutritional support or for the longer term or even for life. Examples include; short bowel syndrome, acute or chronic motility conditions, microvillous inclusion disease, protracted diarrhoea of infancy and Crohn's disease[14,19].

Unlike PN in adults, the nutritional requirements will vary depending on the age of the child to match the demands for growth and development as well as those associated with acute illness. However as in neonates and adults, PN is only indicated if adequate enteral feeding cannot be tolerated[20, 21].

Guidelines on PN in infants and children have been published by the European Society of Paediatric Gastroenterology, Hepatology and Nutrition (ESPGHAN), the European Society for Clinical Nutrition and Metabolism (ESPEN) and the European Society of Paediatric Research (ESPR)[14].

Of the 70 children included in this study the age ranged from one month to 19 years with a median age of eight years. Approximately half the children were cared for in an intensive care or high dependency setting (33/70). The overall quality of PN care for children was found to be slightly better than that in adults and neonates with 24/70 judged to have received good care, however that still leaves 45/70 who received care graded by the Advisor as less than 'good practice'.

The Advisors assessed that there had been adequate consideration for enteral feeding in the majority of children (62 cases) and that the indications for PN were appropriate (62 cases). There tended to be a greater multidisciplinary approach in making the decision to commence PN compared to that in neonatal practice with involvement of nutrition teams in just under half of children (24/57 cases). Surprisingly the adequacy of the initial biochemical and nutritional assessments was judged to be less good (18 cases) compared to that with neonates and this was particularly so in relation to micro biochemical investigations. There was evidence of a nutrition team being involved in 40 cases of children in determining the PN requirements. Furthermore where it could be determined in 41/45 of children the PN was considered adequate for their needs.

The Advisors considered that there was an adequate frequency and level of senior review of ongoing PN (59 cases) but in a quarter of children biochemical monitoring was not adequate (14 cases). Metabolic complications occurred in 10/70 children. The majority of children were weaned onto enteral feeds (48 cases).

In this limited review of PN care of children there is evidence of suboptimal care. While there was greater multidisciplinary PN care with involvement of nutrition teams there were instances of poor initial assessments and inadequate biochemical monitoring. Metabolic complications were apparent.

A large scale national audit of PN care in children should be undertaken.

Case Studies

Adult Case Studies

Case 1

A patient underwent a Hartmann's procedure for a perforated diverticulum. Post-operatively the patient was unable to feed enterally for ten days. On the tenth day a decision was made to initiate PN. However it took a further four days for a feeding catheter to be inserted. In total the patient went without nutrition for 14 days.

Problems identified by Advisors:
1) Delayed recognition of the need for PN.
2) Lack of timely catheter insertion for PN.

Learning points:
1) Patients should not be left for long periods of time without adequate nutrition.
2) Early decision making is necessary to avoid prolonged starvation.
3) Once the decision to start PN is made it should be initiated without undue delay.

Case 2

A very elderly patient with advanced oesophageal cancer and tumour extension through their oesophageal stent was given PN for three days prior to their predictable death.

Problems identified by Advisors:
Advanced carcinomatosis should not be treated with PN.

Learning points:
Whilst PN may appropriate in a very small group of patients who are undergoing palliative care it should generally not be given to this group of patients unless a formal multidisciplinary nutritional assessment has taken place with appropriate palliative care input. The patient should not be moribund.

Case 3

A patient was admitted with total dysphagia secondary to food bolus obstruction. They required an urgent endoscopy to remove the bolus but this was not performed for eight days. Whilst awaiting their endoscopy the patient was given PN.

Problems identified by Advisors:
The patient should have had emergency endoscopy to remove the bolus thus avoiding the need for PN.

Learning points:
PN should not be given as a supporting measure when access to an inaccessible gut can be readily established with urgent intervention. The patient was exposed to the inherent metabolic risks of eight days of PN and a feeding catheter when an endoscopy would have resolved the problem on the day of admission and probably allowed immediate discharge.

Case 4

A patient was recovering from upper gastrointestinal surgery and developed dysphagia. They were started on PN as it was considered that the patient would pull out a nasogastric tube. After PN was commenced they were then referred for a PEG. The gastroenterologist who reviewed the patient considered that they should have had a trial of nasogastric (NG) feeding first.

Problems identified by Advisors:

PN was inappropriate and a trial of NG feeding prior to a PEG would have represented better management.

Learning points:

PN should not be used as a convenience or interim nutritional measure. It should only be used when all forms of enteral feeding have been actively excluded or are impracticable.

Case 5

A female patient with a gynaecological malignancy was treated by pelvic surgery to debulk the tumour. The day following surgery she was able to drink. The surgical team started PN as they found her albumin to be 21g/dL and on the basis of this considered she required nutritional supplementation.

Problems identified by Advisors:

1) There was no indication for PN.

Learning points:

1) If a patient is able to drink then they are likely to be able to take sip feeds and slowly build up their diet.
2) Albumin is a very poor marker of nutritional status and should not be used in the decision to commence PN.

Neonatal and Paediatric Case Studies

Case 6

An extreme low birth weight infant (540g) was born at 26 weeks post-conceptional age. An umbilical venous catheter (UVC) was inserted on the first postnatal day. A radiograph indicated that the tip of the catheter was in right ventricle. The catheter was pulled back 2.5 cm but the position of the catheter was not rechecked until day 3 from birth and was still found to be "too high". The catheter was further withdrawn 1.5 cm. A further radiograph showed "good" position of tip of the catheter. PN was started on day four. There was no attempt at enteral feeding.

Problems identified by Advisors:

1) Poor management of UVC.
2) Poor documentation of UVC insertion and catheter manipulations.
3 No attempt at enteral feeding was made.
4 There was undue delay in starting PN.

Learning points:

1) Insertion of the UVC should have been clearly documented.
2) There should have been expedient verification and action on the position of UVC tip.
3) Nutritional support for this extremely low birth weight infant should have been commenced early following birth.

Case 7

A baby born at 25 weeks post-conceptional age (454g) was commenced on enteral feeding on day 2 from birth. During the next 7 days there was poor absorption of these feeds with bile aspiration from the NG tube. A decision to start PN was made on day 5 but was not started until day 8 to due an intervening weekend. There was low amino acid and lipid content of the initial PN.

Problems identified by Advisors:

1) There was a delay in starting adequate nutritional support with poor recognition of inadequate enteral feeding.
2) The start of PN was delayed after the decision to commence it.
3) There were inadequate constituents of the initial PN.

Learning points:

1) Greater consideration should have been given for this ELBW infant for nutritional support.
2) While it was appropriate to have a trial of enteral feeding there should have been earlier recognition of its failure and PN should been started as soon as possible and at full nutritional value.

Case 8

A baby born at 33 weeks post-conceptional age (2.35 kg) had a laparotomy for duodenal atresia on day 1 from birth. Following surgery an attempt at nasogatric (NG) feeding was made on day 4 from birth. However there were large NG aspirates. Peripheral PN was commenced with low amino acid and lipid content for 10 days. Multiple attempts of PIC catheter insertion were made during this time without success. On day 14 from birth there was still inadequate enteral absorption and the infant had abdominal distension. A contrast abdominal radiograph showed small bowel obstruction. A further laparotomy was performed which revealed a malrotation. A Hickman catheter was inserted at the same time. PN commenced with full nutritional value postoperatively. The infant lost 0.85 kg during the intervening period.

Problems identified by Advisors:

1) There was delayed commencement of full PN.
2) The cause of the prolonged NG losses was not recognised.
3) There was considerable weight loss.

Learning points:

1) The cause of the enteral malabsorption should have been recognised early
2) While it was appropriate to have a trial of enteral feeding there should have been earlier recognition of its failure and PN should have been started as soon as possible and at full nutritional value.

Case 9

A baby born at 29 weeks post-conceptional age with a birth weight of 1.1 kg was admitted to a Neonatal unit for respiratory distress syndrome and suspected sepsis. A PIC catheter was inserted which was clearly documented using a proforma which included a pictorial representation of the site of CVC insertion. The PN was clearly prescribed and was of full nutritional value. The infant was weaned onto full enteral feeding on day 10 after birth.

Learning points:

The Advisors considered that this was an example of both good documentation of catheter insertion and catheter care.

Adult Outcome Data

This study was not designed with the primary aim of looking at outcomes but rather at the quality of care around the administration of PN. However some outcome data were collected. The outcomes for the adult patients and mortality associated with particular indications for PN can be seen in the following tables.

Adult patient outcomes

Outcome	Number of patients
Weaned onto oral/enteral feeds	279
Died during hospital stay	215
Weaned and discharged home	129
Discharged home	113
Transferred	40
Other	16
Home PN	12
Weaned, Transferred	10
Not answered	11
Total	**825**

PN indication and outcome

PN Indication	Alive	Deceased
Post-operative ileus	153	33
Post-surgical complications	95	25
Obstruction	86	24
Non functioning gut	65	35
Failure of enteric nutrition	55	47
Perforated/leaking gut	64	22
Other	53	24
No indication documented	54	10
Fistulae	36	7
No access for enteral nutrition	27	17
Cancer	16	8
Dysphagia	16	8
Malabsorption	13	8
Short bowel	18	4
Dysmotility	13	7
Infection	10	8
Crohn's disease	14	1
Pre-operative nutrition	11	2
Radiation enteritis	5	1
Chemotherapy	6	0
Total	**600**	**214**

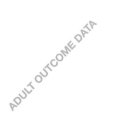

The number of deaths among the adult study group
was 215/814 patients. This is somewhat axiomatic as
it illustrates that patients who require PN are very sick
with an intrinsic disease process and thus have a high
mortality. However, the number of days that PN was given
appears to have little correlation with mortality. The death
rate appears fairly constant across these groups with a
marginally lower mortality in those receiving PN for greater
than 28 days.

PN duration and outcome

	Patient outcome		
Number of Days PN received	**Alive**	**Deceased**	**Total**
1 – 14	432	157	589
15 – 28	62	22	84
>28	41	12	53
Total	**535**	**191**	**726**

NCEPOD suggests that all medical staff are educated
that the administration of inpatient PN is an indicator that
a patient is critically ill and requires close physiological
and biochemical monitoring.

References

1. Organisation of Food and Nutritional Support in Hospitals. BAPEN.2007. www.bapen.org.uk

2. Nutritional support in adults: oral nutritional support, enteral tube feeding and parenteral nutrition. Clinical Guideline (CG)32. NICE.2006. Published by the National Collaborating Centre for Acute Care.

3. British Consensus Guidelines on Intravenous Fluid Therapy for Adult Surgical Patients (GIFTASUP) http://www.bapen.org.uk/pdfs/bapen_pubs/giftasup.pdf

4. American Academy of Pediatrics, Committee on Nutrition: Nutritional needs of low-birth-weight infants. Pediatrics 1977;60:519-30

5. Nutritional needs for Low-Birth-Weight Infants Committee on Nutrition Pediatrics 1985;75:976-86

6. Enteral Nutrient Supply for Preterm Infants: commentary from ESPGHAN. Journal of Pediatric Gastroenterology and Nutrition 2010;50:1-9

7. Growth and development of an infant receiving all nutrients exclusively by vein. Wilmore DW, Dudrick SJ. JAMA 1968;4:860-86

8. Wilson DC, Cairns P, Halliday HL, et al. Randomised controlled trial of an aggressive nutritional regimen in sick very low birthweight infants. Arch Dis Child Fetal Neonatal Ed 1997;77:F4-11

9. Thureen PJ, Melara D, Fennessey PV, Hay WW JR. Effect of low versus high intravenous amino acid intake on very low birth weight infants in the early neonatal period. Pediatr Res 2003;53:24-32

10. Ibrahim H, Jeroudi MA, Baier RJ, Dhanireddy R, Krouskop RW. Aggressive Early Total Parental Nutrition in Low-Birth-Weight Infants Journal of Perinatology 2004;24:482-86

11. Ehrenkranz RA. Early, Aggressive Nutritional Management for Very Low Birth Weight Infants: What Is the Evidence? Semin Perinatol 2007;31:48-55

12. Lapillonne A, Fellous L, Mokthari M, Kermorvant-Duchemin E. Parenteral Nutrition Objectives for Very Low Birth Weight Infants: Results of a National Survey. Journal of Pediatric Gastroenterology and Nutrition 2009;48:618-62

13. Ahmed M, S Irwin S, Tuthill DP Education and evidence are needed to improve neonatal parenteral nutrition practice. J Parenter Enteral Nutr 2004;28: 176-79

14. Koletzko B, Goulet O, Hunt J, et al. Guidelines on Paediatric Parenteral Nutrition of the European Society of Paediatric Gastroenterology, Hepatology and Nutrition (ESPGHAN) and the European Society for Clinical Nutrition and Metabolism (ESPEN), Supported by the European Society of Paediatric Research (ESPR). J Pediatr Gastroenterol Nutr 2005;41(Suppl 2):S1-87

15. Sneve J, Kattelmann K, Ren C, Stevens DC. Implementation of a multidisciplinary team that includes a registered dietician in a neonatal intensive care unit improved nutrition outcomes. Nutr Clin Prac 2009;23:630-34

16. Kuzman-O'Reilly B, Duenas ML, Greecher C, Kimberlin L, Mujsce D, Miller D, Walker DJ. Evaluation, development and implementation of potentially better practices in neonatal intensive care nutrition Pediatrics (2003);111(4):e461-70

17. Robertson's Textbook of Neonatology. Ed J Rennie. 2005;ISBN 0 443 07355 4:3-13

18. Mauro Pittiruti, Helen Hamilton, Roberto Biffi, John MacFie, Marek Pertkiewicz. ESPEN Guidelines on Parenteral Nutrition: Central Venous Catheters (access, care, diagnosis and therapy of complications), Clinical Nutrition 2009;28:4, 365-77

19. Managing children and adolescents on parenteral nutrition: challenges for the nutritional support team. Tracey Johnson T, Sexton E Proceedings of the Nutrition Society 2006;65:217–21

20. Nutrition Therapy in Critically Ill Infants and Children. Heather E. Skillman HE, Wischmeyer PE. J Parenter Enteral Nutr 2008;32:520

21. Guidelines for the Use of Parenteral and Enteral Nutrition in Adult and Pediatric Patients JPEN J Parenter Enteral Nutr. 2002;26(1 Suppl):1SA-138SA

Appendices

Appendix 1 – Glossary

Anthropometric measurement	Mid-arm circumference, tricep circumference and skin fold thickness
Bespoke bags	PN bags tailored to a particular patients' need
Cannulation devices (venous)	A flexible hollow tube, inserted with a guide needle into a vein
Crystalloid	Aqueous solutions of mineral salts and other water soluble molecules e.g. saline
Colloid	Colloids are similar to crystalloid but contain larger soluble molecules such as gelatine
Enteral feeding	The state of being fed by a tube
Extravasation	The accidental administration of intravenously infused fluids into the surrounding tissue
FY	Foundation year doctor
Hypo/hyperglycaemia	Low/High blood sugar
Hypo/hyperkalaemia	Low/High plasma potassium levels
Hypo/hypermagnesaemia	Low/High serum magnesium levels
Hypo/hyperphophataemia	Low/High phosphate levels
Hypo/hypernatraemia	Low/High salt levels
Iatrogenic	Induced inadvertently during by medical treatment of diagnostic procedure
Level 1-3	Level 1 is a ward, Level 2 is a High Dependency Unit and Level 3 is intensive care
Macrobiochemical	PN constitution
Microbiochemical	Electrolytes and vitamins
Micronutrient	Minerals needed in the diet in very small quantities such as iron or zinc
Nasogastric	A tube placed into the stomach via the nose
Nasojejunal	A tube placed into the small bowel (jejunum) via the nose
NCCG	Non consultant career grade doctor
NEC	Necrotising enterocolitis, is a medical condition primarily seen in premature infants where portions of the bowel undergo necrosis (tissue death)
Neonate	A newborn baby or a baby in it's fist 28 days of life
Oedema	An accumulation of fluid beneath the skin or in body cavities
Parenteral nutrition	The state of feeding a person intravenously
Phlebitis	Inflammation of a vein
RFS	Re-feeding syndrome consists of metabolic disturbances that occur as a result of reinstitution of nutrition to patients who are severely malnourished
SAS	Staff and Associate Specialist doctor (includes those previously defined as NCCG doctors above)
ST2	Specialist Trainee doctor Level 2
ST3	Specialist Trainee doctor Level 3
Thrombosis	The formation of a blood clot inside a blood vessel

Appendix 2 – Corporate structure and role of NCEPOD

The National Confidential Enquiry into Patient Outcome and Death (NCEPOD) is an independent body to which a corporate commitment has been made by the Medical and Surgical Colleges, Associations and Faculties related to its area of activity. Each of these bodies nominates members on to NCEPOD's Steering Group.

The Role of NCEPOD

The role of NCEPOD is to describe the gap between the care that should be delivered and what actually happens on the ground. In some ways it is a glorious anachronism: an exercise by the professions themselves to criticise the care that they deliver in the cause of improving the quality of the service provided.

The process is simple but effective. We begin with an idea. Subjects can be suggested by anyone, but most come from the professional associations. It is measure of how deeply the medical profession are committed to the improvement of their service that they should be voluble and enthusiastic about having the care that they deliver assessed and criticised by their peers.

We have far more proposals than we can carry out and each year studies are chosen by competitive secret ballot of the NCEPOD Steering Group, after what is often a lively and partisan debate. In November 2007, when *Parenteral Nutrition* (PN) was chosen with *Surgery in the Elderly* which we will publish later this year, there were a further 12 disappointed studies.

Having gained Steering Group approval, the staff and Co-ordinators together with an Expert Group work up the study design so as to get the raw material that they think they will need to explore the quality of care. They identify a given group of cases and design the study and the questionnaires.

The NCEPOD Local Reporters – our precious eyes and ears in every Trust - are then asked to identify all the cases falling within that cohort. We then send all the Consultants responsible for the cases a questionnaire and elicit the key data that we need. We also ask the Trusts for copies of the notes.

Our staff then go through the notes laboriously anonymising them so that that the Advisors and Co-ordinators cannot identify the patient, the hospital or the staff involved. Inevitably from time to time a perspicacious Advisor will recognise a colleague's handwriting, or even a case from their own hospital: they are trusted to quietly replace it on the pile and draw another.

The Advisors are specialists in the areas of the study but they are emphatically not members of the Expert Group and play no part in the design of the study. They may have no prior connection with NCEPOD but wish to contribute to the over-riding aim of improving care in their specialty. They are trained, being put through dummy runs together with our Co-ordinators, so as to develop the necessary consistency of approach. Their assessment of the cases is done in our premises, in group meetings. Most cases will only be read by one Advisor who fills in an assessment form, but they work together and discuss striking features as they come across them, so that the finished report and the vignettes do not represent idiosyncratic opinions. As you can see from our Acknowledgements they are a multidisciplinary group of distinguished professionals and the final report is compiled by the Co-ordinators and our staff from the material and the judgements made by them for which we are deeply grateful.

Steering Group as at 24th June 2010

Dr R Birks	Association of Anaesthetists of Great Britain and Ireland
Mr T Bates	Association of Surgeons of Great Britain & Ireland
Mr J Wardrope	College of Emergency Medicine
Dr S Bridgman	Faculty of Public Health Medicine
Professor R Mahajan	Royal College of Anaesthetists
Dr A Batchelor	Royal College of Anaesthetists
Dr B Ellis	Royal College of General Practitioners
Ms M McElligott	Royal College of Nursing
Dr T Falconer	Royal College of Obstetricians and Gynaecologists
Mrs M Wishart	Royal College of Ophthalmologists
Dr I Doughty	Royal College of Paediatrics and Child Health
Dr R Dowdle	Royal College of Physicians
Professor T Hendra	Royal College of Physicians
Dr M Clements	Royal College of Physicians
Dr S McPherson	Royal College of Radiologists
Mr B Rees	Royal College of Surgeons of England
Mr M Parker	Royal College of Surgeons of England
Mr D Mitchell	Faculty of Dental Surgery, Royal College of Surgeons of England
Dr M Osborn	Royal College of Pathologists
Ms S Panizzo	Patient Representative
Mrs M Wang	Patient Representative

Observers

Mrs C Miles	Institute of Healthcare Management
Dr R Hunter	Coroners' Society of England and Wales
Dr N Pace	Scottish Audit of Surgical Mortality
Dr K Cleary	National Patient Safety Agency
Ms R Brown	National Patient Safety Agency
Professor P Littlejohns	National Institute for Health and Clinical Excellence

NCEPOD is a company, limited by guarantee
(Company number: 3019382) and a registered charity
(Charity number: 1075588), managed by Trustees.

Appendix 3 – Supporting organisations

The organisations that provided funding to cover the cost
of this study:

National Patient Safety Agency on behalf of the
Department of Health in England and the Welsh Assembly
Government
Department of Health, Social Services and Public Safety
in Northern Ireland
Aspen Healthcare Ltd
BMI Healthcare
BUPA Cromwell
Classic Hospitals
Covenant Healthcare Ltd
East Kent Medical Services Ltd
Fairfield Independent Hospital
HCA International
Hospital of St John and St Elizabeth
Isle of Man Health and Social Security Department
King Edward VII's Hospital Sister Agnes
Netcare Healthcare UK Ltd
New Victoria Hospital
Nuffield Health
Ramsay Health Care UK
Spire Health Care
St Anthony's Hospital
St Joseph's Hospital
States of Guernsey Board of Health
States of Jersey, Health and Social Services
The Benenden Hospital Trust
The Horder Centre
The Hospital Management Trust
The London Clinic
The London Oncology Clinic
Ulster Independent Clinic

DISCLAIMER
This work was undertaken by NCEPOD, which received funding for this report from the National Patient
Safety Agency. The views expressed in this publication are those of the authors and not necessarily those
of the Agency.

Appendix 4 – Trust participation

Trust Name	Number of participating sites within the Trust	Number of clinician questionnaires sent	Number of clinician questionnaires returned	Number of sets of case notes returned	Number of organisational questionnaires sent	Number of organisational questionnaires returned
Aintree Hospitals NHS Foundation Trust	1	18	14	5	1	1
Airedale NHS Trust	1	15	8	7	1	1
Alder Hey Children's NHS Foundation Trust	1	33	21	14	1	1
Aneurin Bevan Local Health Board	2	48	15	8	2	2
Ashford & St Peter's Hospital NHS Trust	1	36	23	29	1	1
Aspen Healthcare	1	-	-	-	1	1
Barking, Havering & Redbridge University Hospitals NHS Trust	2	38	29	28	2	2
Barnet and Chase Farm Hospitals NHS Trust	2	4	3	1	2	2
Barts and The London NHS Trust	2	48	15	7	2	2
Basildon & Thurrock University Hospitals NHS Foundation Trust	1	29	20	18	1	1
Bedford Hospital NHS Trust	1	11	11	11	1	1
Belfast Health and Social Care Trust	3	12	5	3	3	3
Betsi Cadwaladr University Local Health Board	2	23	6	4	2	2
Birmingham Children's Hospital NHS Foundation Trust	1	34	11	3	1	1
Birmingham Women's Healthcare NHS Trust	1	10	10	10	1	1
Blackpool, Fylde and Wyre Hospitals NHS Foundation Trust	1	39	19	36	1	1
BMI Healthcare	11	1	1	0	11	8
Bolton Hospitals NHS Trust	1	22	6	2	1	1
Bradford Teaching Hospitals NHS Foundation Trust	1	19	19	18	1	1
Brighton and Sussex University Hospitals NHS Trust	3	23	15	17	3	3
Buckinghamshire Hospitals NHS Trust	2	24	24	24	2	2
Burton Hospitals NHS Foundation Trust	1	15	15	15	1	1

Trust participation (continued)

Trust Name	Number of participating sites within the Trust	Number of clinician questionnaires sent	Number of clinician questionnaires returned	Number of sets of case notes returned	Number of organisational questionnaires sent	Number of organisational questionnaires returned
Calderdale & Huddersfield NHS Foundation Trust	2	51	41	38	2	2
Cambridge University Hospitals NHS Foundation Trust	1	56	20	6	1	1
Cardiff and Vale University Local Health Board	1	27	15	12	1	1
Central Manchester University Hospitals NHS Foundation Trust	4	25	11	5	4	4
Chesterfield Royal Hospital NHS Foundation Trust	1	12	8	7	1	1
City Hospitals Sunderland NHS Foundation Trust	1	19	19	19	1	1
Clatterbridge Centre for Oncology NHS Trust	1	1	1	1	1	1
Colchester Hospital University NHS Foundation Trust	2	10	7	4	2	2
Countess of Chester Hospital NHS Foundation Trust	1	6	3	1	1	1
County Durham and Darlington NHS Foundation Trust	2	20	9	2	2	2
Cwm Taf Local Health Board	2	19	8	5	2	2
Derby Hospitals NHS Foundation Trust	2	20	18	16	2	2
Doncaster and Bassetlaw Hospitals NHS Foundation Trust	2	41	15	10	2	2
Dorset County Hospital NHS Foundation Trust	1	18	16	18	1	1
Dudley Group of Hospitals NHS Trust	1	21	11	6	1	1
East Kent Hospitals University NHS Foundation Trust	3	57	21	11	3	3
East Kent Medical Services	1	-	-	-	1	1
East Lancashire Hospitals NHS Trust	1	15	6	6	1	0
East Sussex Hospitals NHS Trust	2	31	19	11	2	2
Epsom and St Helier University Hospitals NHS Trust	3	23	10	6	3	3
Frimley Park Hospitals NHS Trust	1	24	16	5	1	1
Great Ormond Street Hospital for Children NHS Trust	1	7	7	7	1	1
Harrogate and District NHS Foundation Trust	1	4	4	2	1	0

Trust participation (continued)

Trust Name	Number of participating sites within the Trust	Number of clinician questionnaires sent	Number of clinician questionnaires returned	Number of sets of case notes returned	Number of organisational questionnaires sent	Number of organisational questionnaires returned
HCA International	4	35	11	10	4	4
Health & Social Services, States of Guernsey	1	5	3	0	1	0
Heart of England NHS Foundation Trust	3	43	17	7	3	3
Heatherwood & Wexham Park Hospitals NHS Foundation Trust	2	8	5	5	2	2
Hereford Hospitals NHS Trust	1	16	16	14	1	1
Hillingdon Hospital NHS Trust	1	20	14	12	1	1
Hinchingbrooke Health Care NHS Trust	1	4	2	1	1	1
Homerton University Hospital NHS Foundation Trust	1	13	6	5	1	0
Hull and East Yorkshire Hospitals NHS Trust	2	8	5	0	2	0
Hywel Dda Local Health Board	3	16	13	13	3	3
Imperial College Healthcare NHS Trust	3	78	26	19	3	3
Ipswich Hospital NHS Trust	1	17	11	11	1	1
Isle of Man Department of Health & Social Security	1	7	5	5	1	0
Isle of Wight NHS Primary Care Trust	1	21	13	10	1	0
James Paget Healthcare NHS Trust	1	10	8	6	1	1
Kettering General Hospital NHS Trust	1	7	6	1	1	1
King's College Hospital NHS Foundation Trust	1	61	15	12	1	1
Kingston Hospital NHS Trust	1	15	13	10	1	1
Lancashire Teaching Hospitals NHS Foundation Trust	2	14	4	2	2	0
Leeds Teaching Hospitals NHS Trust (The)	2	90	39	23	2	2
Lewisham Hospital NHS Trust	1	21	21	18	1	1
Liverpool Heart and Chest Hospital NHS Trust	1	8	3	1	0	0
London Clinic	1	22	1	0	1	1
Luton and Dunstable Hospital NHS Foundation Trust	1	16	5	4	1	1
Maidstone and Tunbridge Wells NHS Trust	2	30	15	4	2	2

Trust participation (continued)

Trust Name	Number of participating sites within the Trust	Number of clinician questionnaires sent	Number of clinician questionnaires returned	Number of sets of case notes returned	Number of organisational questionnaires sent	Number of organisational questionnaires returned
Mayday Health Care NHS Trust	1	12	4	1	1	1
Mid Cheshire Hospitals NHS Trust	1	15	9	6	1	1
Mid Staffordshire NHS Foundation Trust	1	11	6	4	1	1
Mid Yorkshire Hospitals NHS Trust	2	30	24	27	2	2
Mid-Essex Hospital Services NHS Trust	2	26	18	15	2	2
Milton Keynes Hospital NHS Foundation Trust	1	18	9	6	1	1
Newcastle upon Tyne Hospitals NHS Foundation Trust	4	56	42	30	4	4
Newham University Hospital NHS Trust	1	9	5	4	1	1
Norfolk & Norwich University Hospital NHS Trust	1	6	4	4	1	0
North Bristol NHS Trust	2	24	17	16	2	2
North Cumbria Acute Hospitals NHS Trust	2	31	7	6	2	0
North Middlesex University Hospital NHS Trust	1	13	7	1	1	1
North Tees and Hartlepool NHS Foundation Trust	2	30	20	6	2	2
North West London Hospitals NHS Trust	2	13	12	13	2	2
Northampton General Hospital NHS Trust	1	15	9	9	1	1
Northern Devon Healthcare NHS Trust	1	15	11	7	1	1
Nottingham University Hospitals NHS Trust	2	63	38	34	2	2
Nuffield Health	1	-	-	-	1	1
Oxford Radcliffe Hospital NHS Trust	3	52	48	41	3	3
Papworth Hospital NHS Foundation Trust	1	10	8	7	1	1
Pennine Acute Hospitals NHS Trust (The)	3	50	30	26	3	3
Peterborough & Stamford Hospitals NHS Foundation Trust	1	5	5	3	1	1

Trust participation (continued)

Trust Name	Number of participating sites within the Trust	Number of clinician questionnaires sent	Number of clinician questionnaires returned	Number of sets of case notes returned	Number of organisational questionnaires sent	Number of organisational questionnaires returned
Plymouth Hospitals NHS Trust	1	25	18	18	1	1
Poole Hospital NHS Foundation Trust	1	12	9	8	1	0
Portsmouth Hospitals NHS Trust	1	19	4	3	1	1
Princess Alexandra Hospital NHS Trust	1	17	14	6	1	1
Queen Victoria Hospital NHS Foundation Trust	1	-	-	-	1	1
Ramsay Health Care UK	3	-	-	-	3	2
Royal Berkshire NHS Foundation Trust	1	24	21	10	1	1
Royal Bournemouth and Christchurch Hospitals NHS Trust	1	13	8	6	1	0
Royal Brompton and Harefield NHS Trust	2	16	8	5	2	2
Royal Cornwall Hospitals NHS Trust	1	27	23	17	1	1
Royal Devon and Exeter NHS Foundation Trust	1	31	31	31	1	1
Royal Free Hampstead NHS Trust	1	16	15	15	1	1
Royal Liverpool & Broadgreen University Hospitals NHS Trust	1	26	14	14	1	1
Royal Marsden NHS Foundation Trust (The)	2	17	11	9	2	2
Royal Surrey County Hospital NHS Trust	1	23	23	22	1	1
Royal United Hospital Bath NHS Trust	1	23	23	15	1	1
Salford Royal Hospitals NHS Foundation Trust	1	21	10	5	1	1
Salisbury Foundation NHS Trust	1	24	24	24	1	1
Sandwell and West Birmingham Hospitals NHS Trust	2	4	4	4	2	2
Sheffield Children's NHS Foundation Trust	1	6	0	0	1	0
Sheffield Teaching Hospitals NHS Foundation Trust	3	48	27	27	3	3
Sherwood Forest Hospitals NHS Trust	1	19	11	12	1	1

Trust participation (continued)

Trust Name	Number of participating sites within the Trust	Number of clinician questionnaires sent	Number of clinician questionnaires returned	Number of sets of case notes returned	Number of organisational questionnaires sent	Number of organisational questionnaires returned
Shrewsbury and Telford Hospitals NHS Trust	2	33	29	14	2	2
South Devon Healthcare NHS Foundation Trust	1	11	9	8	1	1
South Eastern Health & Social Care Trust	1	12	3	3	1	1
South London Healthcare NHS Trust	3	21	12	3	3	2
South Tees Hospitals NHS Foundation Trust	1	27	27	27	1	1
South Tyneside NHS Foundation Trust	1	14	12	9	1	1
South Warwickshire General Hospitals NHS Trust	1	7	1	0	1	1
Southampton University Hospitals NHS Trust	2	77	53	40	2	2
Southend University Hospital NHS Foundation Trust	1	18	9	7	1	1
Southern Health & Social Care Trust	2	30	9	5	2	2
Southport and Ormskirk Hospitals NHS Trust	1	13	7	5	1	1
Spire Healthcare	9	7	5	1	9	8
St Anthony's Hospital	1	-	-	-	1	1
St George's Healthcare NHS Trust	1	3	3	3	1	0
St Helens and Knowsley Teaching Hospitals NHS Trust	1	18	18	18	1	1
Stockport NHS Foundation Trust	1	-	-	-	1	1
Surrey & Sussex Healthcare NHS Trust	1	17	17	15	1	1
Tameside Hospital NHS Foundation Trust	1	12	9	8	1	0
Taunton & Somerset NHS Foundation Trust	1	17	17	17	1	1
The Christie NHS Foundation Trust	1	20	14	10	1	1
The Rotherham NHS Foundation Trust	1	13	8	12	1	1
Trafford Healthcare NHS Trust	1	2	0	0	1	1
University Hospital of South Manchester NHS Foundation Trust	1	3	1	1	1	0

Trust participation (continued)

Trust Name	Number of participating sites within the Trust	Number of clinician questionnaires sent	Number of clinician questionnaires returned	Number of sets of case notes returned	Number of organisational questionnaires sent	Number of organisational questionnaires returned
University College London Hospitals NHS Foundation Trust	1	26	12	6	1	1
University Hospital Birmingham NHS Foundation Trust	1	15	11	11	1	1
University Hospitals Coventry and Warwickshire NHS Trust	1	22	22	22	1	1
University Hospitals of Bristol NHS Foundation Trust	2	54	44	34	2	2
University Hospitals of Leicester NHS Trust	3	47	35	35	3	3
University Hospitals of Morecambe Bay NHS Trust	2	32	31	23	2	2
Velindre NHS Trust	1	4	4	4	1	1
Walton Centre NHS Foundation Trust	1	2	0	0	1	0
Warrington & Halton Hospitals NHS Foundation Trust	1	-	-	-	1	1
West Middlesex University Hospital NHS Trust	1	12	4	0	1	1
West Suffolk Hospitals NHS Trust	1	23	22	22	1	1
Western Health & Social Care Trust	1	27	18	17	1	1
Western Sussex Hospitals NHS Trust	3	39	26	22	3	3
Whipps Cross University Hospital NHS Trust	1	17	17	16	1	1
Whittington Hospital NHS Trust	1	11	11	6	1	1
Winchester & Eastleigh Healthcare NHS Trust	1	13	4	2	1	1
Wirral University Teaching Hospital NHS Foundation Trust	1	21	15	9	1	1
Worcestershire Acute Hospitals	2	31	16	7	2	2
Wrightington, Wigan & Leigh NHS Foundation Trust	1	4	4	3	1	1
Yeovil District Hospital NHS Foundation Trust	1	5	1	1	1	0
York Hospitals NHS Foundation Trust	1	13	11	9	1	1

Trusts/hospitals from which no data were recevied and for which no reason was provided

Barnsley Hospital NHS Foundation Trust
Basingstoke & North Hampshire Hospitals NHS Foundation Trust
Chelsea & Westminster Healthcare NHS Trust
Dartford & Gravesham NHS Trust
Ealing Hospital NHS Trust
East & North Hertfordshire NHS Trust
East Cheshire NHS Trust
Gateshead Health NHS Foundation Trust
George Eliot Hospital NHS Trust
Gloucestershire Hospitals NHS Foundation Trust
Great Western Hospitals NHS Foundation Trust
Guy's & St Thomas' NHS Foundation Trust
Hospital of St John and St Elizabeth
King Edward VII's Hospital Sister Agnes
Liverpool Women's NHS Foundation Trust
Medway NHS Foundation Trust
New Victoria Hospital
Northern Health & Social CareTrust
Northern Lincolnshire & Goole Hospitals Trust
Northumbria Healthcare NHS Foundation Trust
Queen Elizabeth Hospital NHS Trust
Queen Mary's Sidcup NHS Trust
Robert Jones and Agnes Hunt Orthopaedic & District Hospital
Royal National Orthopaedic Hospital NHS Trust
Royal Orthopaedic Hospital NHS Foundation Trust
Royal Wolverhampton Hospitals NHS Trust (The)
Scarborough and North East Yorkshire Health Care NHS Trust
South Downs Health NHS Trust
States of Jersey Health & Social Services
The Horder Centre
The London Oncology Clinic
The Queen Elizabeth Hospital King's Lynn NHS Trust
Ulster Independent Clinic
United Lincolnshire Hospitals NHS Trust
University Hospital of North Staffordshire NHS Trust
Walsall Hospitals NHS Trust
West Hertfordshire Hospitals NHS Trust
Weston Area Health NHS Trust